This book constitutes the first systematic attempt to bring together the vast field of postmodern and post-structuralist nursing literature from the late 1980s through the first decade of the 2000s. Olga Petrovskaya demonstrates this literature's significant contribution to "theorizing nursing" in a mode of *critique*. *Critique* here refers to analyses attentive to historicity, materiality, and politics of nursing practice and nursing knowledge. She contrasts this with the mostly American literature on "nursing theory," construed mainly in terms of formal systematization. Her main argument is that the American understanding of "nursing theory" has dominated nursing textbooks across the globe, to the extent that the many modes of "theorizing nursing" are rendered mostly invisible. She raises important questions about how these two almost radically opposed conceptualizations of theory and their methods and/or status in nursing qua knowledge influence what is taught to and studied by nursing students and scholars. The work is highly original in scope and depth and should be considered required reading for all nursing scholars.

– Miriam Bender, PhD, RN, FAAN
Associate Professor
Founding Director, Center for Nursing Philosophy
Sue & Bill Gross School of Nursing
University of California, Irvine

There's a lot to be written about the history of academic nursing theory, and this is a hefty contribution to our understanding of one prominent slice of it. Olga Petrovskaya has written an intriguing analysis of American nursing scholarship, and the way in which its parochialism, self-celebration, *ex officio* nursing values, and old-fashioned positivism preclude serious consideration of postmodern and poststructuralist ideas, rendering them largely unintelligible to U.S. nurses. Petrovskaya describes American theory's three responses to French philosophy, Foucault in particular. Ignore it. Dismiss it. Assimilate a domesticated, housebroken version of it. And she suggests that this is consistent with the ideal of an isolationist "unique nursing science" – its drawbridge up, its portcullis down – freezing out any challenge to its canon from other philosophies, other disciplines, other parts of the world. Perhaps this book will turn out to be the unstoppable force that dislodges the hitherto immovable object of American nursing theory. That could be a watershed moment. But this is American nursing theory. I'm not holding my breath.

– John Paley,
University of Worcester

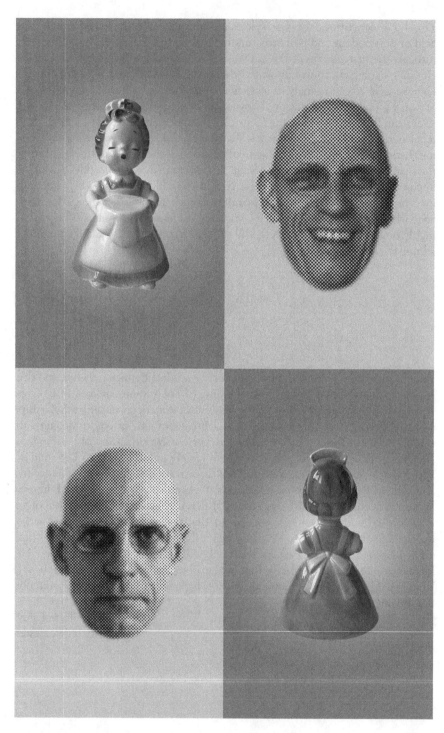

Figure 0.1 It's Not About Being Comfortable Bedfellows

Source: Bogdan Shablya

Nursing Theory, Postmodernism, Post-structuralism, and Foucault

Nursing Theory, Postmodernism, Post-structuralism, and Foucault critiques mainstream American nursing theory and its use of post-structural theory, comparing and contrasting how postmodern and post-structural ideas have been used fruitfully in nursing research and theorizing elsewhere.

In the late 1980s, references to post-structuralism and Michel Foucault started to appear in nursing journals. Since then, hundreds of nursing publications have cited postmodernism and key post-structural ideas such as power/knowledge, discourse, and de-centring the human subject. In *Nursing Theory, Postmodernism, Post-structuralism, and Foucault*, Olga Petrovskaya argues that the application of these ideas is markedly different in American nursing theory scholarship compared to nursing theoretical scholarship generated outside the canon of "unique" nursing theory. Analysing relevant literature from the late 1980s through 2010s, she demonstrates this difference, arguing that American nursing theory calcified into a matrix of dogmas built on logical positivism, wary of "borrowed" theory, and loyal to a "unique nursing science." Post-structural ideas that fit the matrix, such as criticism of medicine, are sanctioned, whereas ideas sceptical of humanistic agendas including those that challenge American nursing theory are rendered meaningless. In contrast, other nurse scholars from Britain, Australia, Canada, and what the author calls the American enclave group engaged with postmodern and post-structural perspectives to enrich their research and invite readers to rethink nursing practice. The book showcases examples of their intelligent, creative theorizing. Arguing that American nursing theory enervated nursing theorizing, Petrovskaya calls for opening this matrix to theoretical and methodological creativity, less rigid categories of scholarship, and healthy self-examination.

Making the case that post-structural ideas are vital for nurses' ability to critically reflect on their discipline and profession, this is a necessary read for all those interested in nursing theory, philosophy, and praxis.

Olga Petrovskaya is an assistant professor in the University of Victoria School of Nursing in British Columbia, Canada. She is an active and long-standing member of the International Philosophy of Nursing Society (IPONS), and in 2021 she was elected to serve as the vice chair of IPONS. Dr. Petrovskaya is interested in continental philosophy especially German critical theory and French post-structuralism as well as a contemporary direction in social theory called *practice theory*. In 2014 she won first prize in the *Nursing Philosophy* journal Graduate Student Writing Contest for her article, "Is There Nursing Phenomenology after Paley?" Dr. Petrovskaya's funded program of research combines her interest in eHealth and Health Information and Communication Technology with her interest in theoretical perspectives attuned to the socio-materiality of health care practices, for example, actor network theory. She teaches undergraduate and graduate courses on nursing knowledge and theory development.

Routledge Research in Nursing and Midwifery

A Theory of Cancer Care in Healthcare Settings
Edited by Carol Cox, Maya Zumstein-Shaha

Motherhood, Spirituality and Culture
Noelia Molina

Joy at Birth
An Interpretive, Hermeneutic, Phenomenological Inquiry
Susan Crowther

Paradoxes in Nurses' Identity, Culture and Image
The Shadow Side of Nursing
Margaret McAllister and Donna Lee Brien

Birthing Outside the System
The Canary in the Coal Mine
Edited by Hannah Dahlen, Bashi Kumar-Hazard and Virginia Schmied

Nursing and Humanities
Graham McCaffrey

Grading Student Midwives' Practice
A Case Study Exploring Relationships, Identity and Authority
Sam Chenery-Morris

Complexity and Values in Nurse Education
Dialogues on Professional Education
Edited by Martin Lipscomb

Nursing Theory, Postmodernism, Post-structuralism, and Foucault
Olga Petrovskaya

For more information about this series, please visit:
www.routledge.com/Routledge-Research-in-Nursing/book-series/RRIN

Nursing Theory, Postmodernism, Post-structuralism, and Foucault

Olga Petrovskaya

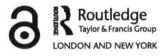
Routledge
Taylor & Francis Group
LONDON AND NEW YORK

First published 2023
by Routledge
4 Park Square, Milton Park, Abingdon, Oxon OX14 4RN

and by Routledge
605 Third Avenue, New York, NY 10158

Routledge is an imprint of the Taylor & Francis Group, an informa business

© 2023 Olga Petrovskaya

British Library Cataloguing-in-Publication Data
A catalogue record for this book is available from the British Library

Library of Congress Cataloging-in-Publication Data
A catalog record has been requested for this book

ISBN: 978-1-032-04728-7 (hbk)
ISBN: 978-1-032-34320-4 (pbk)
ISBN: 978-1-003-19443-9 (ebk)

DOI: 10.4324/9781003194439

Typeset in Goudy
by Apex CoVantage, LLC

Contents

Foreword   viii
Acknowledgements   xii

1   Early 21st-Century Canadian Nursing at a Theoretical
    Crossroads: Between American Nursing Theory and
    British-Australian Post-structural Theorizing   1

2   Establishing the Field of Study: Postmodern, Post-
    structural, and Foucauldian Nursing Scholarship   20

3   American Nursing Science and Discipline-Specific
    Theory: In the Grips of Logical Positivism   38

4   Postmodern and Post-structural Ideas in American
    Nursing Texts I: Gortner, Dzurec, Reed, Watson, and
    Nursing Science Quarterly   58

5   Postmodern and Post-Structural Ideas in American
    Nursing Texts II: *Advances in Nursing Science* and the
    Enclave Group   82

6   Postmodern and Post-structural Ideas in Non-American
    Nursing Literature: Examining Nurse–Patient
    Relationships and the Holistic Nurse   102

7   It's Not About Being Comfortable Bedfellows: Why
    Postmodern and Post-structural Literacy Matters in Nursing   120

Appendix   139
Index   169

Foreword

by Mary Ellen Purkis
Professor Emerita, School of Nursing, University of Victoria

While nurses are often characterized as struggling to attain legitimacy in the academy, around the health policy table, and at the patient's bedside, they have too rarely drawn on a critical examination of the knowledges informing their practices as a way of advancing their professional interests. Indeed, as Petrovskaya argues in this excellent volume, concern with the relationship between knowledge and practice has been woefully underexamined. Entering into this field to explore this interesting state of affairs, Petrovskaya presents the reader with a clear and critical assessment of the dominant discourses that have had an overweighted influence on organizing the field of nursing knowledge. She examines the contours of those discourses, exposing both the framing of knowledge as well as its effects. She also exposes the distinct, even paradigmatic edges – paradigmatic in that colloquial sense of solving problems internal to the discourse but "unintelligible" to other framings of knowledge.

There are three concepts given detailed treatment in this book, which I would like to focus my comments on: knowledge, practice, and theory. What stands out for me in reading this text is the underlying concern for *practice* that has been raised again and again throughout nursing's intellectual development. Petrovskaya draws our attention to that concern in introducing readers to the pioneering work of Susan Gortner. Gortner is widely credited with leading the establishment of this new field of inquiry that quickly became known as nursing science. Emerging from the post-war years, nursing had gained a strongly positive reputation certainly in its important *relationship* to medicine but also independently with reference to its *unique and distinct practices* supporting patients through illness and in their return to health. There were, no doubt, specific reasons why nursing developed as a particular sort of professional force in the United States through the 1950s and 1960s. And perhaps it was the turmoil of those years, the frenetic energy fuelling numerous fields of knowledge and research, nursing being one among many, that even someone of Gortner's stature could not hold the focus of this burgeoning profession on that concept of practice. Gortner's leadership as a newly minted nurse scientist was to shine a light on the relationship of the nurse's knowledge and its effects – through nursing practice – on patients.

But as Petrovskaya's history of ideas illustrates, instead, American nurse academics, for the most part, chose a different path. They set an interest in practice aside in favour of theory – aspirational, conceptual, and quite decontextualized from the concerns and interests of practicing nurses. For those of us who entered into schools of nursing in North America in the 1970s and beyond, it was common to learn that faculty members had selected a particular theory to guide the induction of new recruits into the profession. The organizing features of such theories afforded students a useful frame upon which to attach the multiple new experiences encountered in the world of hospital-based nursing practice. Those features offered concepts and themes for faculty members to organize lectures and activities for students entering hospital wards – and, in return, they enabled students to produce work aligned with those concepts and themes in order to demonstrate themselves – ourselves! – as well-organized students, capable of becoming registered nurses.

This very practical effect of a focus on theory, the training of recruits, is rarely noted in the discipline's theoretical commentary – perhaps one more way in which those North American nurse academics have been blind to practice. This represents one of many clear illustrations of Petrovskaya's argument regarding a deep and profound *unintelligibility* between the dominant set of ideas organizing nursing knowledge by North American nurse academics versus the less well-organized but interesting ideas that were beginning to frame discourses of knowledge in nursing from other sociogeographic locations. Petrovskaya does note the ways in which North American nursing theory was practiced in schools of nursing in the United States and Canada. In doing so, she opens the possibility for readers that clear separations between knowledge, theory, and practice as required by the traditions of North American theory developers might not be necessarily so separate. In fact, allowing practice and theory and knowledge to play together was beginning to produce some important and interesting insights into nursing's place in the academy and in the clinic.

The theme of conflict between theory and practice arises several times as Petrovskaya takes readers through nursing's history of ideas. For instance, it arises again in Chapter 3 where key thinkers of the day propose completely opposing prescriptions for the discipline's support of a full academic role for itself. Due to Petrovskaya's careful curating of these ideas, we can see that at the same time that Dorothy Johnson and Rozella May Schlotfeldt were recommending that the discipline of nursing should articulate and guide an agenda for research and theory development that would then be tested in practice, other leaders in academic nursing – who has not heard of Dickoff and James in this context? – were proposing that researchers should await the appearance of problems in practice and use those to drive research that would solve those problems. Echoes of Susan Gortner's exhortations are found in this debate.

But these conflicts have never been so clearly articulated to enable debate on different ways to develop knowledge for the discipline. This is one of the key contributions of this volume. Petrovskaya shows us that those conflicting views have often been softened through re-formulation and incorporation into the body of theoretical writings – as though the conflicts were of no consequence. The possibility that knowledge developed from problems encountered in practice may be of a radically different sort than knowledge imposed on practice from a particular set of philosophical ideas arising far away from practice – and from a stance that, at the time, treated practice as acontextual as well as ahistorical, is neither contemplated nor examined in those earlier writings.

And so, this book will pose significant challenges to that largely settled history of nursing's intellectual development as established in the dominant literature promulgated by North American nursing academics. In the latter third of the text, Petrovskaya shines a light on a pathway less well explored in North America but well established now by British, Australian, European, and Canadian scholars. Again, seeking to show that the relationship between practice, theory, and knowledge matters, she draws on authors whose work has troubled the boundaries of geographically established understandings of these relationships. She shows us what it means, and how we have to alter our own established thinking and practicing – whether in the clinic or in our academic work – when we adopt poststructuralist ideas such as the decentred subject and anti-humanism. Nursing is a discipline and profession that has, for so long, deeply entwined its understandings of itself on the centrality of the person/patient in order to gain access to a mind that is viewed as propelling the body in health and illness and therefore a mind and body to be influenced towards particular versions of health by professional care workers. Tying its scholarly traditions to humanistic frames born of the Enlightenment has unnecessarily contracted the discipline and the knowledges it could draw on to better understand the relationships between practitioners and those they seek to help.

And this is where my commentary will end with a strong encouragement to readers to delve into these interesting and exciting ideas that Petrovskaya presents, with a return to my three concepts of knowledge, practice, and theory.

I do so by referencing the work of Alfred Schütz, writing in 1946 – again, at that time of expanding and confusing ideas following World War II. Schütz offers an interesting perspective on the nature of knowledge and how we can think about it being shared amongst citizens where modern life is characterized by a strong conviction that the individual's "life-world as a whole is neither fully understood by himself (sic) nor fully understandable to any of his fellow-men (sic)" (p. 463). Through the intervening eight decades this experience of modern life holds. Despite the repetitive character of an 8- or a 12-hour shift, each shift brings something new to light for the nurse who demonstrates an interest in their practice. The situation of the nurse, according to Schütz, is to adopt what he calls "socially approved knowledge" or "socially derived knowledge." Both forms accept that knowledge is socially distributed. Knowledge is not inherent in the knowing subject but rather is apprehended *as knowledge* and adopted either on the basis of powerful influences (e.g. socially approved knowledge) or on the basis of critique of the interests at play in the formation of knowledge (e.g. socially derived knowledge).

Petrovskaya's volume offers readers an engagement in the history of ideas in nursing in the tradition of Schütz's socially derived knowledge. For Schütz, socially approved and socially derived knowledge are understood as being in constant interplay. What Schütz calls the *natural attitude* or *taken-for-granted world of everyday life* represents an important enabling feature for all social beings as we move through every day. Schütz recognized that we cannot and do not continuously second guess every move we make before we make it, every statement made by others, every action taken independently or in concert with others. Instead, "the relatively natural concept of the world from which all inquiry starts and which all inquiry presupposes, reveals itself as the sediment of previous acts of experiencing – my own as well as that of others – which are socially approved" (p. 478). In seeking to examine the interests coalescing around socially approved knowledge, one is bound to raise questions that those in positions of authority prefer to leave settled. Disrupting settled knowledge may at times be noisy and create alarm – but if we follow Schütz, engaging in a careful and systematic study of those ideas is critical to a healthy and robust science in an open society. This volume offers just such an exemplary study.

Reference

Schütz, A. (1946). The well-informed citizen: An essay on the social distribution of knowledge. *Social Research, 13*(1), 463–478.

Acknowledgements

This book grew out of my dissertation. Over the years, many individuals and scholarly groups sparked my initial and ongoing interest in the topic of nursing theory and nursing philosophy. Regardless of how these scholars positioned their own work, they helped me, wittingly or otherwise, articulate my arguments in the book. Some of these scholars would not necessarily share my viewpoint or even recognize the issues discussed in this book, but I believe that one of the best things that can happen to an academic is to have an intelligent opponent.

In my PhD in nursing program at the University of Victoria, Canada, Dr. Mary Ellen Purkis inspired and supported my interest in the work of Michel Foucault and in social theory and introduced me to the members of In Sickness and In Health (aka the "Foucauldian group" of international nurse scholars). I still benefit from Mary Ellen's wise mentorship that started with her encouraging supervision of my dissertation work more than a decade ago. Another University of Victoria scholar and a member of my supervisory committee, Dr. Anne Bruce, was a kind, patient, and thoughtful reader of many drafts. Anne's intellectual generosity and respect for diverse scholarly genres is exceptional. Dr. Stephen Ross from the English department and the interdisciplinary "Cultural, Social, and Political Thought" program was instrumental to my engagement with the French philosophy of post-structuralism. If I failed to do justice to all the intricacies of postmodernism and post-structuralism as these are known in the humanities and social sciences, this is purely my fault, perhaps reflective of nursing's often peculiar ways of taking these philosophies on board.

During my early PhD years, Drs. Marjorie McIntyre and Carol McDonald introduced me to the American post-structural queer theorist Judith Butler. At that time, a momentous event happened: I learned about the International Philosophy of Nursing Society (IPONS) and started attending its annual conferences. Further, the Banff philosophy conferences organized by the Unit for Philosophical Nursing Research (uPNR) at the University of Alberta became the must-attend scholarly events for me. The works of numerous fine scholars I met at those and other conferences are cited throughout the book: Sioban Nelson, Davina Allen, Christine Ceci, Trudy Rudge, Kristin Bjornsdottir, Joanna Latimer, John Paley, John Drummond, and Gary Rolfe. A special place among them is occupied by Mark Risjord, an analytic philosopher of science. Although far removed from and often sceptical of "the French theory," his work on nursing science plays a significant role in my analysis in the book. Mark, John Paley, and Derek Sellman deserve a special mention for reading my entire dissertation and sharing their comments when I was contemplating its publication some time ago. Martin Lipscomb described his positive experiences with Routledge, which finally nudged me to proceed.

My heartfelt thank-you goes to Dr. Madeline Walker, an editor, a poet, and a gentle friend, whom I praise for helping to strengthen my English language skill. Madeline is an intelligent reader who "gets" the topic of nursing theory! Her able editorial and research support made this book possible. If at times I still use long sentences and express convoluted ideas, it is because my native language conventions are hard to fully suppress.

I am indebted to my husband, who supported my book through tireless behind-the-scenes work of keeping the household going while I spent long days at my desk. A heartfelt thank-you to my son who created the artistic image the reader discovers upon opening the book.

The University of Victoria and my academic unit have supported aspects of my work on the book through the much-appreciated Book Subvention fund and Dorothy Kergin award.

And last but not least, this work was ably supported by Grace McInnes and Evie Lonsdale, my contacts at Routledge, and I express gratitude for their interest and patience.

1 Early 21st-Century Canadian Nursing at a Theoretical Crossroads

Between American Nursing Theory and British-Australian Post-structural Theorizing[1]

Based on my analysis of the encounter between American nursing theory and French postmodern/post-structural ideas from the late 1980s through the first decade of the 2000s, I argue in this book that American nursing theory appears incapable of grasping the crucial differences between its humanistic assumptions and the theoretical anti-humanism of post-structuralism. Instead, American nursing theory subsumes heterogeneous theoretical perspectives within its established intellectual matrix rendering them bland, acritical, and even meaningless. My intent is not so much to argue for the privileged place of French philosophy in particular but to arrive at the end of the book to ask a question about the future of theorizing in the discipline of nursing. As new important and relevant post-humanist theoretical currents develop in social sciences and humanities and trickle into the nursing literature, will (American) nurse theorists be able to engage with perspectives drastically diverging from and challenging Western humanism?

What follows is my personal reflection about my nursing educational experiences in Canada. I relay how I encountered various nursing theories: ways to *theorize* in the discipline of nursing, or ways to produce particular texts consisting of interconnected sets of ideas for the purpose of describing or explaining (aspects of) nursing and thereby helping us understand nursing practice. These encounters, which also extend beyond the discipline of nursing into the interdisciplinary realm of critical social and political thought, surfaced the jarring incoherence between the two kinds of theorizing referred to in this chapter's title. One, emphatically, is a definition from a nursing text: "Theory – an internally consistent group of relational statements that presents a systematic view about a phenomenon and that is useful for description, explanation, prediction, and prescription or control" (L. O. Walker & Avant, 2011, p. 7). And another, as emphatically, is a speculation from a sociology text: "Social theory . . . is the art, if not always the science, of asking the right questions at the risk of irritating the hell out of those who have already settled the matter to their satisfaction" (Lemert, 2009, p. xvi).

Theory as a formal system and theory as critique: In nursing, I met both. With time I realized, however, that it is only the former kind of theories – those couched in the formal vocabulary of "internal consistency," "relational statements," and

DOI: 10.4324/9781003194439-1

"systematic view" (as in L. O. Walker & Avant, 2011); of "concepts," "propositions," "internal dimensions," and "theory testing" (as in Meleis, 2007); of "concepts," "theoretical assertions," and "logical form" (as in Tomey & Alligood, 2006) or incorporated within Fawcett's (2005) "structure of contemporary nursing knowledge" – that nursing *theory* textbooks recognize as legitimate "disciplinary knowledge." How can this be the case? This quandary set me on the path of my study.

Before elaborating on my theoretical encounters, I sketch the plan for this chapter and provide a map for the whole book where I walk the reader through the chapters that follow and indicate the main lines of argument. This introductory chapter also includes a section on methodological considerations. I suggest that this book might be usefully identified as metatheoretical and that it aims at developing a scoping overview and comparison of nursing literature citing post-structural philosopher Michel Foucault in a specific period from the late 1980s throughout the first decade of the 2000s. I briefly explain theoretical notions like *episteme*, *discourse*, and the *conditions of possibility* originating in Foucault's (1966/1994, 1969/1982) work that helped frame my questions and provided lines for analyses.

Theory's Predicament

During my Canadian undergraduate and master's nursing education in the first decade of the 2000s, I took several classes designed to introduce and ground students in the unique knowledge of our discipline. Course titles invariably referred to *nursing theory* and *nursing knowledge development*. We learned that throughout the 1960s and 1970s American nurse scholars discussed the development of "nursing science" conceived as the body of discipline-specific theories that distinguish nursing knowledge from the biomedical knowledge of physicians. The work of building nursing knowledge over the ensuing decades culminated in an impressive volume of published metatheoretical debates, books authored by individual nurse theorists, and compilations of nursing theories.

Nursing programs at a college and two universities in Toronto, where I was successively enrolled, adopted different nursing theories to guide their curricula. Curriculum of one of the undergraduate programs was based on Sister Callista Roy's adaptation model (Roy, 1988; Roy & Andrews, 1999). This model used concepts from general systems theory to postulate nursing-specific axioms. Roy's model conceptualized humans as holistic, adaptive systems and discussed such a system in terms of inputs (stimuli), outputs (e.g. adaptive responses), and control and feedback process. Having the program's curriculum based on a nursing theory presupposed that the students, when they worked with patients in their clinical placements, would couch clinical nursing observations and patient care plans in the language of that theory.

The other undergraduate program adopted a "caring curriculum" articulated within nursing's human science tradition (Bevis & Watson, 1989). Several nurse scholars in this program self-identified as "Parse scholars," after prominent

American nurse theorist Rosemarie Rizzo Parse. Again, students' analyses of clinical encounters ("self-reflective narratives") were to be written through the conceptual lens of Parse's humanbecoming theory (Cody & Mitchell, 2002; Jonas-Simpson, 1997; Mitchell & Cody, 1992, 2002; Parse, 1996, 1997). However, the master's program employed a different curricular approach. Critical of grounding a graduate curriculum in a specific nursing theory or philosophy, the program of study nevertheless included a course on nursing theoretical developments, with quite rigorous and challenging assignments.

As the reader shall see in Chapter 3, the phrase *nursing theory* came to signify in American literature, as well as beyond, a set of theories formulated mostly throughout the 1970s and 1980s[2] – the theories said to comprise the content of *unique nursing disciplinary knowledge*. Some thinkers see these theories as a progressive step of building a nursing science in the academy. A more sceptical perspective (e.g. Davina Allen, 1998; Dingwall & Davina Allen, 2001; May & Fleming, 1997; May & Purkis, 1995; see also Nelson, 2003) sees this disciplinary theory-building work as struggles for power and status in the social arena, a "professionalization project," a dissatisfaction of nursing's elite members with nursing's occupational status and their struggle to gain a more influential role for nurses in health care. American nurse scholars have envisioned a nursing science broader than the natural sciences, or, more precisely, broader than "empiricist medical science." This breadth is variably signalled through multiple "patterns of knowing" articulated in our discipline: aesthetic, personal, and ethical in addition to empirical (Carper, 1978), sociopolitical (White, 1995), and emancipatory (Chinn & Kramer, 2008, 2015); multiple "paradigms" (e.g. Fawcett, 2005; Newman, 1992; Newman et al., 1991; Parse, 1987), and the view of nursing as a human science (e.g. Mitchell & Cody, 1992).

In the 1960s and 1970s, several influential nurse scholars believed that the autonomy of the nascent discipline of nursing in the academy depended on its status as a unique nursing science. Aligned with the dominant mid-20th century philosophy of science, a unique nursing science presupposed abstract theories that neither offer prescriptions for clinical practice nor draw directly from other disciplines. In other words, a conception of science embraced by many (but not all) in American nursing theoretical literature dictated that these theories were neither practically useful for everyday work nor did they conform to theoretical formulations common within other disciplinary fields. (This conception of nursing science is presented in Chapter 3.) Thus, "borrowed" theories were to be treated with caution. Even more comprehensive nursing knowledge textbooks that included chapters on theories from other disciplines (e.g. McEwen & Wills, 2007) left no doubt about the distinction: "Borrowed theory" is to be unambiguously separated from nursing's "unique knowledge." It was only in my doctoral program that I discovered another kind of theorizing, in both nursing and interdisciplinary milieus.

Conferences and networks (most notably, International Philosophy of Nursing Society, *In Sickness and In Health*, and Philosophy in the Nurses' World conferences) I attended as a doctoral student were energizing venues for theorizing, where critique of current political, professional, and practical realities of nursing flourished. The nurse scholars discussed theory, research, and philosophy; clearly, they were engaged in the development of nursing knowledge. The relevance of these understandings *of* practice and their potential *for* informing nursing practice was tangible. Yet, this theoretical discourse did not correspond to the image of theory and theoretical knowledge upheld by the American nursing metatheoretical literature. Most notably, this newly discovered form of scholarship boldly drew on "borrowed theory" (often of an anti- and post-humanist kind) without caution: French post-structural theory, science and technology studies, and selected sociological theory. Remarkably, these intellectual tools were used in an unsettling way to examine and critique not only the realities of nursing practice but often the very assumptions of American nursing science and theory (e.g. David Allen, 2006; Ceci, 2003; Drevdahl, 1999a; D. Holmes & Gastaldo, 2002; Latimer, 2000; Lawler, 1991a; May & Purkis, 1995; Nelson, 1995, 2000; J. Parker, 2004a, 2004b; Rudge, 1998; Traynor, 1996).

Curiously, attending the conferences I noticed that besides several Canadian academics, the nursing networks interested in postmodern and post-structural theory included scholars from the United Kingdom and some other European countries, as well as Australia, but rarely from the United States. However, through reading, I learned that in the 1990s, an American-led group organized the International Critical and Feminist Perspectives in Nursing conferences.[3] A portion of Chapter 5 brings to the reader's attention a small constellation of interesting postmodern and post-structural American nursing publications, produced by what I call the "enclave group" – nurse scholars participating in the Critical and Feminist Perspectives conferences, several of whom were connected to the University of Washington nursing program.

The majority of nursing scholarship informed by postmodern and post-structural theory, however, has been produced outside the United States, most notably by Australian and New Zealand, British and Irish, and Canadian scholars.[4] In Chapter 6, I acknowledge the diversity of this work and then focus on two early examples of nursing post-structural scholarship: theorizing of the nurse–patient relationship (May, 1990, 1992a, 1992b, 1995a, 1995b) and a history of the holistic nurse (Nelson, 2000).

These primarily British and Australian nurses and/or social scientists interested in nursing practice have read a French post-structural philosopher, Michel Foucault, to show how his work contested the established conceptions of history, subjectivity, humanism, power, language, and meaning and how these critiques are relevant for nursing. They analysed nursing practice in its contextual and historical complexity. These authors experimented with postmodern approaches to research. In short, selected non-American postmodern and post-structural nursing writings described in Chapters 6 mobilize a Foucauldian ideal of *thinking* – reflection upon limits (Ceci, 2013) – or in other words, a critical reflection of the discipline on itself.

Returning from the nursing philosophy conferences and delving into the textbooks on nursing theory featuring Roy's adaptation model, Jean Watson's caring theory, or Peggy Chinn's integrated model for knowledge development, I struggled to make sense of the different ways that the notion of *theory* was taken up in the conference papers versus the way it was dealt with in American nursing theory textbooks.

My educational experience as a nursing student in Canada is not representative of all Canadian nursing programs. Courses on nursing theory and nursing knowledge development are included in the curricula of many, but not all, nursing programs. I was taught by some prominent Canadian scholars who obtained their doctoral degrees in the United States. They studied with influential nurse theorists and continued to shape the tradition in Canada. Although academic nursing in the United Kingdom and Australia was less swayed by North American nursing's disciplinary developments, metatheoretical literature on nursing science and nursing theory reached those locales. Some nurse academics from Australia and the United Kingdom passionately objected to the imposition of American-style nursing theory onto their respective educational fields (Drummond, 2013; C. Holmes, 1991; Lawler, 1991b) and practice settings (Mason & Chandley, 1990) or patiently analysed the assumptions and implications of the new models and demonstrated their problematic features (Davina Allen, 1998; Cribb et al., 1994; Dingwall & Davina Allen, 2001; Latimer, 1995; May, 1990; Traynor, 1996). Other Australian and British nurse academics embraced various American theoretical formulations (e.g. selected authors in Gray & Pratt, 1991; McKenna, 1997; McKenna & Slevin, 2011; Murphy & C. Smith, 2013). Over the decades, American nursing theory has expanded its sphere of influence. A unique disciplinary "structure of nursing knowledge" similar to Fawcett's (2005) was even envied by an Irish nurse academic (McNamara, 2010) in the context of the transition of nurse preparation in Ireland to an educational sector. Generally, however, the presence of nursing theory – and more importantly, of explicit philosophies of science driving the development of nursing theory and the associated understanding of "nursing knowledge" – was the strongest in the United States and Canada.

Curiously, the modes of theorizing displayed in the philosophy nursing conferences I enjoyed were similar to those I observed elsewhere, outside the discipline of nursing, in the theoretically oriented humanities and the interpretive social sciences. That is, nurse-Foucauldians shared a language with the interdisciplinary social theorists, but this language was somehow inadequate to participate in the discourses of *nursing theory*. What I heard at the conferences seemed to align with my experience of reading post-structural writings within humanities and social science courses, but increasingly it was becoming apparent that it was the theory presented within the nursing classroom that did not seem to speak either to the nursing scholarship presented at the (theory- and philosophy-rich) conferences or to the post-structural scholarship presented in the humanities or social science literature I was exposed to. In other words, theory as it is presented in the nursing classroom and circulated through influential American textbooks is relatively isolated. Differences in "technical" conceptual repertoires of nursing theory versus social theory (e.g. Foucault-based work) can only go so far to explain this observation. That some nurse writers operated with the terms like *postmodernism* and *post-structuralism*, to which others were not privy, was not the whole story explaining the lack of translatability between (mostly non-American) post-structural nursing theorizing and the discourse of American nursing theory. After all, as Chapters 4 and 5 establish, some American nurse theorists have cited Foucault and written about "postmodernism." Rather, as I aim to demonstrate in this book, American theoretical discourse has developed (within) particular understandings of the framework of nursing knowledge and its proper elements, for example, metaparadigm, paradigm, levels of theory, and a vision of unique nursing science sealed off from interdisciplinary theory. Theoretical pronouncements lacking these elements are unintelligible as a kind of *nursing knowledge*, even when concerned with an apparently mutually relevant subject matter, for example, a nurse–patient encounter. This raised a question for me (Petrovskaya et al., 2019): Do not perceptive analyses of nursing practice written outside of the canon of American nursing theory exemplify nursing theory/ theorizing and philosophizing that enrich the knowledge base of the discipline? An article by Purkis and Bjornsdottir (2006) is a good example of theorizing nursing practice, yet, due to the prescriptive format imposed by the American theoretical matrix that fills our textbooks, it is considered outside of the realm of nursing theory.

In "Intelligent Nursing: Accounting for Knowledge as Action *in* Practice," Purkis and Bjornsdottir (2006) offer an alternative view of a contested notion of "nursing knowledge," arguing for the limitations of conceptions of nursing knowledge foregrounded by the prominent and polarized perspectives: evidence-based practice and (or vs.) nurse's intuitive and emotional knowing amplified by her healing potential as a human being (Petrovskaya et al., 2019). To do this, Purkis and Bjornsdottir examine a scenario from a field study of home care nursing. A theoretical notion of *competing temporalities* from the work of J. Parker, an Australian nurse who draws on postmodern ideas and insights from the social studies of science, forms a basis for the analysis of the scenario. The participants in the home care situation – the patient, nurse, physician, and health care system – are teased apart and shown as "embedded in diverse temporalities" (Purkis & Bjornsdottir, 2006, p. 253) that create challenges for "being in the same moment" for various actors. The ever-present ambiguities of practice are shown to emerge in a *particular spatiotemporal context* and can only be negotiated *there*. But what is most important, from the authors' point of view, is an understanding of *context* and of what they call dual activation: Ethical and effective nursing practice – intelligent practice – demands that the nurse be *activated* by different forms of knowledge and that she *activates*, or establishes, "a context for nursing care *through* knowledge" (Purkis & Bjornsdottir, 2006, p. 255; italics in original). "In cooperation with the patient options are explored and the rules within which they encounter one another are set" (p. 255). Purkis and Bjornsdottir offer an understanding of "the operations of knowledge in the practice of nursing" (p. 248), operations that happen outside "the modernist temporality directed towards the future" (Parker, 1997, quoted in Purkis & Bjornsdottir, 2006, p. 247).

Arguably, this analysis is a fine case of nursing theory, of philosophizing nursing practice, of enabling the nurse reader to see and think their familiar everyday realities and struggles from a different vantage point – a shift that might open spaces for nurses' ethical, practical negotiations in situ without a promise of attaining transcendence or a heightened moral ground that some nursing theory valorizes (Petrovskaya et al., 2019). Yet, against the background of American nursing theory and "unique" disciplinary literature, Purkis and Bjornsdottir's (2006) work – its style, methodology, and even the world of nursing practice, though painfully recognizable – is unintelligible as the domain of "proper nursing knowledge." At best, it counts as an important addition to the "unique knowledge" of nurses, an optional supplement that can help an autonomous nurse to appreciate the "peripheral" context of practice.[5]

It is not that continental philosophy does not figure in American nursing textbooks and journals. Indeed, critical social theory and phenomenology/hermeneutics have been embraced as "alternative paradigms" of unique nursing science. Staring from the late 1990s, some American nursing science/theory texts (Chinn & Kramer, 2004, 2011; Meleis, 2007, 2012; Polifroni & Welch, 1999; Reed & Shearer, 2009; Rodgers, 2005) expanded their domain to include postmodernism and post-structuralism. However, this process was selective and uneven. Continental ideas were characteristically transformed to fit the established intellectual matrix. In Chapter 4, I examine several anthologized and thus better-known American "postmodern" articles. My analysis in that chapter aims to surface specific mechanisms through which the discourses of nursing science and nursing theory enable and constrain French-informed thought. Overall, in Chapters 4 and 5, I set out an argument that within the American theoretical nursing literature, postmodern and post-structural nursing theorizing remained largely invisible and as if unreadable within the prevailing intellectual matrix.[6]

In a sense, my argument in this book reflecting the first two decades of nursing's encounter with postmodern and post-structural French theory arose from a uniquely Canadian crossroads; I was positioned between the influential body of American nursing theory *and* (primarily non-American) postmodern and post-structural nursing theorizing. I had one foot in the American journals *Nursing Science Quarterly* and *Advances in Nursing Science*, the mighty advocates of nursing theory, while my other foot was in Foucault-dense nursing literature: the British *Journal of Advanced Nursing* (where Foucault was first cited) and the two now-Canadian journals, *Nursing Inquiry* (for several years the utmost forum for Foucauldian scholarship; originally under Australian editorship) and *Nursing Philosophy* (open to diverse philosophical perspectives; originally under British editorship).

From this vantage point, both generative and conflicting, I argue that the wealth of insightful nursing theoretical work informed by postmodern and post-structural ideas has not been recognized as a form of theorizing worthy of the designation, "nursing knowledge." I aim to show how, during the 1990s and into the 2010s, the enduring intellectual matrix of American nursing theory organized and directed nurses' understandings of what constitutes appropriate theory.

This intellectual matrix, namely "unique nursing science" – as well as its product, "nursing theory" – is grounded upon a logical positivist conception of science.[7] Only relatively recently has the magnitude of logical positivist influence on key nursing theoretical ideas been fully and systematically analysed by Mark Risjord (2010). In Chapter 3, I turn to Risjord's critiques and summarize his pertinent points. An exposition of the logical positivist influences on nurses' conception of theory leads to the following conclusion: Understandings of theory and theorizing enabled within the discourse of American nursing science and nursing theory leave certain *continental* theoretical practices (approaches to theorizing, textual products, substantive concerns) outside the matrix of intelligibility of "proper disciplinary knowledge." Or, in other words, American nursing science/nursing theory discourses produce a peculiar *matrix of (in)visibility* (a term I explain later in the chapter) in relation to nursing analyses informed by postmodern and post-structural French thought.

At issue here is not that we should add diverse forms of scholarship to the body of existing American nursing theory. I neither suggest that "nursing theory" makes room for newer forms of theorizing, nor do I propose that continentally inspired theorizing or novel perspectives from the social sciences fit into the existing and discursively dominant "nursing knowledge structure" of one or another ilk. On the contrary, I hope that my ideas can contribute to a re-visioning of the established "structure" itself: interrogation of the understandings that ground American nursing science/theory, including understandings about form, substance, assumptions, and purposes of nursing theory. This re-visioning is necessitated by the realities of clinical nursing practice as historical and social processes and in light of questions raised by nursing's encounter with critical social theory/philosophy (especially its anti- and post-humanist varieties), and by critiques produced in nursing literature (e.g. Davina Allen, 2014; Drevdahl, 1999a, 1999b; Edwards, 2001; Kim & Kollak, 2006; Liaschenko, 1997; Nelson, 2003; Nelson & Gordon, 2004; Paley, 2002, 2006; Risjord, 2010; Thompson et al., 1992) but largely ignored by American nurse theorists. This and other conclusions and implications are pursued in Chapter 7.

Methodological Considerations

Resistant to settling on an unambiguous category of "methodology" in this book, I invite the reader to consider my methodology as metatheoretical textual analyses of nursing literature intentionally scoped for its references to postmodernism, post-structuralism, and/or Foucault and published roughly over the first two decades of this academic field. The rationale for this timeframe is outlined in Chapter 2.

This book continues a relatively long tradition of nurses reflecting on their discipline and the profession – in other words, of nursing's (meta)theoretical scholarship. This tradition goes back at least to the 1950s, when nursing academic publications proliferated in the United States. As all those works do, I am theorizing about theory. I do not seek to examine any particular theory, be it any specific American nursing theory or Foucault's work. Rather, I seek to recast the existing nursing theoretical discourses in light of the following questions: How has postmodern and post-structural thought entered nursing scholarship and evolved through the 1990s and 2000s? What is the relationship between the prevailing disciplinary intellectual matrix embodied by American nursing theory and the *(un)intelligibility* of post-structural thought in nursing, particularly in American nursing literature? What are the conditions that produce the (in) visibility of scholarship drawing on anti-humanist French theory? In other words, the process and the outcome of theorizing in the context of this book mean advancing a critical perspective on the nursing theoretical field.

To respond to these questions, I view nursing disciplinary literature from a historical vista, tracing not only the development of theoretical ideas in nursing (roughly chronologically from the late 1980s into the 2000s as Chapter 2 explains) but also, to some extent, the conditions and effects of their emergence. This task, whenever possible, relies on and is built upon what I came to identify as landmark nursing texts. One such relatively recent critical and well-informed source is *Nursing Knowledge: Science, Practice, and Philosophy* (Risjord, 2010) – a systematic examination of the six-and-a-half decades of the American nursing scientific discourse against the backdrop of the 20th-century debates in the philosophy of science. My own examination of nursing's expressly *non-scientific* terrain inhabited by French theory would have been much more difficult to accomplish without the clarity provided by Risjord's analysis.[8]

I refer interchangeably to scholarship that I examine in my work as postmodern and post-structural, French theory-inspired, Foucauldian, and as adopting the assumptions of theoretical anti-humanism. The basis for such usage will become clear in Chapter 2. Although French thinkers whose work these labels attempt to capture tended to dispute them, I am adopting a term *French theory*, invented in the humanities departments in the United States, to refer to the intellectual current brought from Europe to the United States early in the second half of the 20th century (Cusset, 2008). The watershed moment happened in 1966 when a group of leading French theorists presented their work at Johns Hopkins University (Macksey & Donato, 1970). For better or for worse, this and consecutive exchanges between the French and American academy transformed the social sciences and the humanities in the United States (Cusset, 2008) and elsewhere. Numerous theory textbooks in sociology, political science, English literature, literary criticism, education, and other disciplines reflect those changes. Nurse authors from Australia, Canada, the United Kingdom, the United States, Scandinavian countries, Brazil, and other places also encountered French theory and brought novel ideas to bear on nursing issues.

How did I go about textual analysis? The analysis brought together diverse *nursing* literature: philosophical, both continental and philosophy of science; American nursing theory; social historical; and research methodological sources. I engaged in a close and systematic reading that attended to the historical context of writing (primarily the ideational context in the discipline of nursing and the larger academy), discursive positions occupied by individual authors and whole journals, stylistic and narrative features, networks of textual production and circulation (i.e. citation patterns, links between authors, journal and text-book affiliations, and market longevity of nursing textbooks), and effects that the discourses of unique nursing science generated in American nursing literature and beyond – particular understandings of both critical social theory/philosophy and its nursing counterparts, as well as nurses' practices of teaching and writing. My reading was also comparative and strove to bring together positions and counter-positions that might benefit from cross-exposure. Occasionally, I turned to literature from the humanities and social sciences to contextualize, clarify, or extend a point made in nursing literature.

I read for both *what* texts mean and *how* they mean it. The *what* assumes taking care to understand the author's perspective (which always exceeds the author's intent), while also acknowledging that the text is always recast in light of the question I am posing about/to it. The *how* means paying attention to rhetorical strategies, style, genre, and to the effect of persuasion. In addition, my attitude towards "knowledge" contained in the various sources I examined was coloured by the following insight:

> Truth is a thing of this world: it is produced only by virtue of multiple forms of constraint. And it induces regular effects of power. Each society has its regime of truth, its "general politics" of truth: that is, the types of discourse which it accepts and makes function as true; the mechanisms and instances which enable one to distinguish true and false statements, the means by which each is sanctioned; the techniques and procedures accorded value in the acquisition of truth; the status of those who are charged with saying what counts as true.
>
> (Foucault, 1977/1980a, p. 131)

This attitude invites treating all texts as particular practices of representation and as forms of discourse produced within the webs of power. According to another perspective, analytical procedures should be attuned to three levels of discourse: the micro-level with attention to rhetorical devices and phrases; the level of dominant, marginal, silent, and competing discourses, their functions, and the speaker's positions within; and the level of social and historical context (Fairclough, 1992, cited in Wilson, 2001, p. 297).

It is worth emphasizing that one of the conclusions I made early in the process of reading nursing works citing Foucault was that there is little point in comparing nursing postmodern/post-structural/Foucauldian scholarship with its counterpart in the non-applied fields of the humanities and social sciences. If the interpretation of Foucault in political science and literary studies is held as a litmus test for rigour, similar nursing works will often appear lacking. In contrast, I suggest that comparisons *within* the nursing literature, that is, a comparison between the work of American nurse theorists citing Foucault and Foucault-informed nursing literature generated outside of this canon (and often critical of it) is fair and fruitful.

What I find useful, rather than forcing any specific categorization of the methodology, is to identify specific theoretical notions that triggered my imagination, felt generative throughout the process, and provided optics through which to establish the field of study and view nursing literature: Foucault's notions of the episteme and the conditions of possibility and Butler's notion of intelligibility.[9]

Foucault's Episteme and the Conditions of Possibility

In *The Order of Things*, Foucault (1966/1994) explained his intent to "reveal a *positive unconscious* of knowledge: a level that eludes the consciousness of the scientist and yet is part of scientific discourse" (p. xi; italics in original). Thus, the episteme is "the historical a priori that grounds knowledge and its discourses and thus represents the condition of their possibility within a particular epoch" ("Episteme," Michel Foucault section, para. 1). About a decade later, Foucault (1977/1980b) summarized the notion of episteme thus:

> The strategic apparatus which permits of separating out from among all the statements which are possible those that will be acceptable within . . . a field of scientificity, and which it is possible to say are true or false. The *episteme* is the "apparatus" which makes possible the separation, not of the true from the false, but of what may from what may not be characterised as scientific.
>
> (p. 197)

An apparent change in this latter explanation of the *episteme* (Foucault, 1977/1980b) relates to Foucault's shift to the study of "apparatuses" (an apparatus of sexuality; Foucault, 1976/1978) and "disciplines" (penal system, schools, etc.; Foucault, 1975/1995) in his later work. The notion of apparatus allowed Foucault to pursue his interest in the operations of power (see also Foucault, 1971/1984) without, however, abandoning the *episteme*. That is, he extended his focus from the episteme, knowledge, and discursive formations to *apparatuses*, that is, relationships among heterogeneous elements, both discursive and non-discursive (p. 197). By the "non-discursive," Foucault (1977/1980b) meant "institutions," that is, any system of constraint in a society producing "learned behaviour" (p. 197). Responding to the question of whether the institution is itself discursive, Foucault admitted that his analyses do not rely on neatly distinguishing between the two but rather on accepting their interdependence (p. 198).

The notion of episteme was particularly fruitful for helping me grasp the profound and unrecognized influence that the "structure of nursing knowledge" and the (logical-positivist) conception of theory (e.g. described by Fawcett, 2005, and permeating the American nursing theory field) have had on how French postmodern and post-structural theory was applied in the American theoretical nursing literature. A specific understanding of theory that founds the structure of American disciplinary knowledge (Risjord, 2010) and a specific understanding of the preferred content of American nursing theory as focusing on the ideology of humanism and holism (Nelson, 2000) create the conditions of possibility for what kind of theorizing is accepted as "nursing knowledge."[10]

The Matrix of Intelligibility

A dictionary defines *unintelligible* as impossible to understand ("Unintelligible," *Longman Dictionary*). In the humanities, since the 1990s, this notion acquired notable theoretical importance (Rodriguez, 2011) as a result of work by Judith Butler (1990). Butler, an American philosopher, feminist, and queer theorist, is perhaps best known for her analyses of the social construction of gender. She argues that gendered bodies are understood, made intelligible, against a pervasive cultural background of meanings, a certain signifying system. In the West, "the heterosexual matrix" provides "a grid of cultural intelligibility through which bodies, genders, and desires are naturalized" (Butler, 1990, p. 151). In short, Butler argues that a heterosexual matrix makes only heterosexual bodies intelligible and renders homosexual/queer bodies unintelligible. Using this insight more as an inspiration than direct analogy, I argue that the American nursing theory matrix makes only a certain form of nursing knowledge intelligible, excluding other forms of scholarship as unintelligible. Intelligibility implies access to the subject's inherent nature. That is, when something is considered intelligible, not only is it rendered understandable, its assumed essence is also revealed.

With the publication of Risjord's (2010) critique of the philosophical underpinnings of unique nursing science, it became possible to appreciate the depth and spread of a logical positivist conception of science within the American theoretical field, which stakes a claim on the entire domain of *nursing* knowledge. This historically formed and persistent understanding of "proper disciplinary theory" and "nursing knowledge" creates a matrix within which theoretical/theory-informed scholarship is cast as intelligible or otherwise. The most rigorous iteration of this matrix requires that scholarship proves its *nursingness* through assimilating into the "distinctive body of extant nursing knowledge." One of the most robust insistences on nursingness is Fawcett's uncompromising manifesto:

> I will continue to advocate for using nursing discipline-specific conceptual models and theories as the basis for all practical activities in nursing. . . . I will not work directly with nurses who chose to contribute to other disciplines by using the conceptual models and theories of those other disciplines; nor will I praise their efforts as contributions to advancement of nursing knowledge.
> (Butts, 2012, pp. 153–154)

My use of parentheses in *(un)intelligible* signals a double function of this matrix: legitimizing and assimilating those forms of theorizing that adhere to the formal and rhetorical conventions of this matrix, while keeping invisible and as if unreadable other forms of theoretical scholarship.[11]

Concluding Thoughts

This chapter sets the stage for the exploration of the first two decades of nursing postmodern and post-structural scholarship that unfolds over the next six chapters. My approach – an argument with elements of metatheoretical and comparative textual analyses of the intentionally scoped body of literature – attempts sensitivity to the historical, textual, and cross-disciplinary contexts. I began with an observation of my situatedness at what I depicted as the Canadian nursing theoretical crossroads: being exposed to both American nursing theory and continentally informed nursing theorizing citing postmodern and post-structural theory and written outside the American nursing theory canon. This situation is generative, but it is also contradictory considering American "unique" nursing science's claim that its theories are the exclusive container for nursing knowledge. This claim arises from a conception of nursing science based on unrecognized and lasting influences of a logical positivist philosophy of science. In the American theoretical nursing literature, this dominant intellectual matrix created a double effect – incorporating certain versions of a "postmodern" scholarship while rendering other readings of French theory nearly unintelligible and as if unworthy of the designation nursing knowledge. Outside American nursing science, however, especially in the United Kingdom, Australia, Canada, and internationally, postmodern and post-structural nursing scholarship had taken markedly different forms (e.g. methodological, stylistic) and addressed a wider range of issues, including significant critiques of the assumptions of American nursing theory itself.

Notes

1 As the title implies, and as will be made clear in the book, there is a divergence between conceptions of theorizing (i.e. developing theoretical knowledge) in the American nursing theory literature and elsewhere. *Theory development* in the American nursing theory movement has become a codified activity with an outcome (theory) expected to look a particular way. In nursing literature outside the American nursing theory canon, the term *theory* has a more interdisciplinary connotation, referring to a scientific theory or a literary theory, as well as to American nursing theory. Thus, *theorizing* or a process of describing, explaining, and so on, usually has a broader meaning and more informal character outside the American nursing theory literature. Theorizing, in this broad sense, can include (or can be found in) analyses of the findings of empirical research studies, philosophical nursing papers, or what is often called theoretical discussion papers. In other words, the term *theory* has a rather fixed meaning in the context of academic nursing in the United States, referring to the American nursing theory movement and a plethora of textbooks containing the intellectual product called "theory." In contrast, the term *theorizing* is what I call the process, and it is an outcome of analytical activity reflected in many nursing writings.

2 Textbooks on "nursing knowledge" variously distinguish among frameworks, theories, conceptual models, and philosophies. I use the term *theory* in a broad sense to include all these formulations. American nursing theory textbooks place the beginning of the nursing theory movement in the 1950s (with the work of Peplau, V. Henderson, and others) and the early 1960s (e.g. Orlando, Wiedenbach). However, Risjord (2010)

argues that the appropriation of these early writings into the metadiscourse of unique nursing science/nursing theory happened in the 1970s.

3 These conferences continued in the first decade of the 21st century, but I could locate only scattered records of these activities. As far as I am aware, around 2015, the University of Sydney Faculty of Nursing and Midwifery attempted to revive a tradition of these conferences.

4 I mention Australian, British, and Canadian scholars throughout the book because these authors comprised a majority of postmodern and post-structural writings during the period I studied. However, strictly speaking, this group also includes authors from New Zealand and Ireland.

5 The American nursing theory textbook that included this article is the fifth edition of Reed and Shearer's *Perspectives on Nursing Theory* (2009). Still, Purkis and Bjornsdottir's (2006) paper along with a few other continentally informed articles in this anthology are so thoroughly embedded in the dominant American "structure of nursing knowledge" with its specific concerns and prescriptions for how theory is developed, that I doubt the intelligibility of Purkis and Bjornsdottir's *style and substance of theorizing* – accessible yet using an unfamiliar theoretical angle – among a wider nursing community inculcated into American nursing theory.

6 Needless to say, overall, both American nursing theory *and* nursing continental theorizing as *forms of scholarship* have been outnumbered by less-explicitly theoretical types of research. The latter includes clinically, biomedically focused research as well as various quantitative, qualitative, and mixed-method studies that do not undertake explicitly theoretically, critically grounded analyses. Parenthetically, these kinds of research are also theoretical, albeit in a different way, according to insights from the social studies of science, communication and rhetoric studies, and contemporary philosophy of science – insights presented in nursing literature, for example, by Sandelowski (1993, 2008, 2011) and Risjord (2010).

7 A logical positivist conception of science, as presented by Risjord (2010) and referred to as *logical empiricist conception* by Bluhm (2014) in her own analysis reinforcing that of Risjord, encompasses the following set of beliefs: a pyramid model of science comprised of hierarchical levels of theory from grand to practice theory, based on their level of abstraction; theories as sentences (less-abstract propositions are derived from abstract laws by a process of logical deduction); a number of metaparadigm concepts guiding the development of a scientific field; science encompassing incommensurable paradigms; and scientific disciplines developing unique theories that do not communicate with "borrowed theories" from outside the discipline.

8 This does not suggest, however, that Mark Risjord shares or endorses my book's interest in French philosophies of postmodernism and post-structuralism. He describes his work as an analytic philosophy of science, and I am capitalizing on his lucid analysis of logical positivist influences on American nursing theory. Further argument in my book that compares various postmodern, post-structural, and Foucauldian nursing work neither suggests nor requires Risjord's investment.

9 When combining various philosophical ideas, one should take care to avoid cherry-picking one's examples or texts in a way that betrays the larger systems to which they belong. Foucault's ideas, for example, are only compatible so far with Butler's (or Derrida's, for that matter) before they conflict, so that combining them or using one to expand upon the other may not be coherent. I thank Dr. S. Ross, University of Victoria, for emphasizing this point. Indeed, the issue of cherry-picking is not uncommon in nursing literature. In my earlier publications (Petrovskaya, 2014a, 2014b), I have acknowledged the challenge for nurse scholars – who might not have relevant background – to work with philosophical and theoretical ideas from other disciplines.

10 I avoid drawing a direct parallel between Foucault's (1966/1994, 1969/1982) archaeological work and my project. For example, Foucault (1966/1994) conceived of the

"systems of regularities that have a decisive role in the history of the sciences" (pp. xiii–xiv) on a scale of several sciences (biology, linguistics, and political economy), whereas my project is much more circumscribed.

11 Occasionally, philosopher of science Thomas Kuhn used the phrase "disciplinary matrix" to refer to a constellation of "strong commitment by the relevant scientific community to their shared theoretical beliefs, values, instruments and techniques, and even metaphysics," an explanation synonymous with his chief notion of paradigm (Bird, 2013, "The Development of Science," para. 4). While at a glance this description corresponds to my use of the term *matrix* as a metaphor for American nursing science/nursing theory, I suggest that Foucault's notion of episteme holds a stronger analytical potential for my work. (Besides, the notion of paradigm is a loaded one in both nursing theory and qualitative research.) A similarity between Foucault's episteme and Kuhn's paradigm has been noted by some commentators ("Episteme," Michel Foucault section, para. 4). However, these commentators discerned differences between episteme and paradigm. For example, paradigm-shifts are the result of conscious decisions, whereas episteme often operates as the "epistemological unconscious" or a "positive unconscious of knowledge" (Foucault, 1966/1994, p. xi). Whereas Kuhn posits the dominance of one paradigm within normal science, Foucault searches for possibilities of opposing discourses within a science. I do not claim a relation to or the influence of Kuhn's writings. To recap, a phrase I use, "intellectual matrix of (un) intelligibility," is a nod to Foucault's conception of the episteme (and relatedly, his *conditions of possibility*) and Butler's notions, *matrix* and *intelligibility*.

References

Allen, D. (1998). Record-keeping and routine nursing practice: The view from the wards. *Journal of Advanced Nursing, 27*(6), 1223–1230.

Allen, D. (2006). Whiteness and difference in nursing. *Nursing Philosophy, 7*(2), 65–78.

Allen, D. (2014). Re-conceptualising holism in the contemporary nursing mandate: From individual to organisational relationships. *Social Science & Medicine, 119*, 131–138.

Bevis, E. O., & Watson, J. (Eds.). (1989). *Toward a caring curriculum: A new pedagogy for nursing.* NLN.

Bird, A. (2013). Thomas Kuhn. In E. N. Zalta (Ed.), *The Stanford encyclopedia of philosophy.* http://plato.stanford.edu/entries/thomas-kuhn/

Bluhm, R. L. (2014). The (dis)unity of nursing science. *Nursing Philosophy, 15*(4), 250–260.

Butler, J. (1990). *Gender trouble: Feminism and the subversion of identity* (1st ed.). Routledge.

Butts, J. B. (2012). The future of nursing: How important is discipline-specific knowledge? A conversation with Jacqueline Fawcett. Interview by Dr. Janie Butts and Dr. Karen Rich. *Nursing Science Quarterly, 25*(2), 151–154.

Carper, B. (1978). Fundamental patterns of knowing in nursing. *Advances in Nursing Science, 1*(1), 13–23.

Ceci, C. (2003). Midnight reckonings: On a question of knowledge and nursing. *Nursing Philosophy, 4*(1), 61–76.

Ceci, C. (2013). Analysing and reflecting on limits. *Nursing Philosophy, 14*(3), 151–153.

Chinn, P. L., & Kramer, M. K. (2004). *Integrated knowledge development in nursing* (6th ed.). Mosby.

Chinn, P. L., & Kramer, M. K. (2008). *Integrated theory and knowledge development in nursing* (7th ed.). Mosby Elsevier.

Chinn, P. L., & Kramer, M. K. (2011). *Integrated theory and knowledge development in nursing* (8th ed.). Mosby Elsevier.

Chinn, P. L., & Kramer, M. K. (2015). *Knowledge development in nursing: Theory and process* (9th ed.). Elsevier Health Sciences.

Cody, W. K., & Mitchell, G. J. (2002). Nursing knowledge and human science revisited: Practical and political considerations. *Nursing Science Quarterly, 15,* 4–13.

Cribb, A., Bignold, S., & Ball, S. (1994). Linking the parts: An exemplar of philosophical and practical issues in holistic nursing. *Journal of Advanced Nursing, 20*(2), 233–238.

Cusset, F. (2008). *French theory: How Foucault, Derrida, Deleuze, & Co. transformed the intellectual life of the United States* (J. Fort, Trans.). University of Minnesota Press.

Dingwall, R., & Allen, D. (2001). The implications of healthcare reforms for the profession of nursing. *Nursing Inquiry, 8*(2), 64–74.

Drevdahl, D. (1999a). Sailing beyond: Nursing theory and the person. *Advances in Nursing Science, 21*(4), 1–13.

Drevdahl, D. (1999b). Meanings of community in a community health center. *Public Health Nursing, 16*(6), 417–425.

Drummond, J. S. (2013). John S. Drummond. In A. Forss, C. Ceci, & J. S. Drummond (Eds.), *Philosophy of nursing: 5 questions* (pp. 45–54). Automatic Press/VIP.

Edwards, S. D. (2001). *Philosophy of nursing: An introduction.* Palgrave Macmillan.

Fawcett, J. (2005). *Contemporary nursing knowledge: Analysis and evaluation of nursing models and theories* (2nd ed.). F. A. Davis.

Foucault, M. (1978). *The history of sexuality. Volume 1: An introduction* (R. Hurley, Trans.). Random House. (Original work published 1976)

Foucault, M. (1980a). Truth and power. In C. Gordon (Ed.), *Power/knowledge: Selected interviews and other writings, 1972–1977* (pp. 109–133, Interview with A. Fontana & P. Pasquino). Pantheon Books. (Original work published in French 1977)

Foucault, M. (1980b). The confession of the flesh. In C. Gordon (Ed.), *Power/knowledge: Selected interviews and other writings, 1972–1977* (pp. 194–228). Pantheon Books. (Original work published in French 1977)

Foucault, M. (1982). *The archaeology of knowledge & the discourse on language* (A. M. Sheridan Smith, Trans.). Pantheon Books. (Original work published in French 1969)

Foucault, M. (1984). Nietzsche, genealogy, history. In P. Rabinow (Ed.), *The Foucault reader* (pp. 76–100). Pantheon Books. (Original work published in French 1971)

Foucault, M. (1994). *The order of things: An archaeology of the human sciences.* Vintage Books. (Original work published in French 1966)

Foucault, M. (1995). *Discipline and punish: The birth of the prison* (A. Sheridan, Trans.). Vintage Books. (Original work published in French 1975)

Gray, G., & Pratt, R. (Eds.). (1991). *Towards a discipline of nursing.* Churchill Livingstone.

Holmes, C. (1991). Theory: Where are we going and what have we missed along the way? In G. Gray & R. Pratt (Eds.), *Towards a discipline of nursing* (pp. 435–460). Churchill Livingstone.

Holmes, D., & Gastaldo, D. (2002). Nursing as means of governmentality. *Journal of Advanced Nursing, 38*(6), 557–565.

Jonas-Simpson, C. (1997). Living the art of the human becoming theory. *Nursing Science Quarterly, 10*(4), 175–179.

Kim, H. S., & Kollak, I. (Eds.). (2006). *Nursing theories: Conceptual and philosophical foundations* (2nd ed.). Springer Publishing Company.

Latimer, J. (1995). The nursing process re-examined: Enrollment and translation. *Journal of Advanced Nursing, 22*(2), 213–220.

Latimer, J. (2000). *The conduct of care: Understanding nursing practice.* Wiley.

Lawler, J. (1991a). *Behind the screens: Nursing, somology and the problem of the body*. Churchill Livingstone.

Lawler, J. (1991b). In search of an Australian identity. In G. Gray & R. Pratt (Eds.), *Towards a discipline of nursing* (pp. 211–227). Churchill Livingstone.

Lemert, C. (2009). *Social theory: The multicultural and classic readings* (4th ed.). Westview Press.

Liaschenko, J. (1997). Ethics and the geography of the nurse–patient relationship: Spatial vulnerabilities and gendered space. *Scholarly Inquiry for Nursing Practice, 11*(1), 45–59.

Macksey, R., & Donato, E. (Eds.). (1970). *The structuralist controversy: The languages of criticism and the sciences of man*. Johns Hopkins University Press.

Mason, T., & Chandley, M. (1990). Nursing models in a special hospital: A critical analysis of efficacity. *Journal of Advanced Nursing, 15*(6), 667–673.

May, C. R. (1990). Research on nurse–patient relationships: Problems of theory, problems of practice. *Journal of Advanced Nursing, 15*(3), 307–315.

May, C. R. (1992a). Individual care – power and subjectivity in therapeutic relationships. *Sociology, 26*(4), 589–602.

May, C. R. (1992b). Nursing work, nurses' knowledge, and the subjectification of the patient. *Sociology of Health and Illness, 14*(4), 472–487.

May, C. R. (1995a). "To call it work somehow demeans it": The social construction of talk in the care of terminally ill patients. *Journal of Advanced Nursing, 22*(3), 556–561.

May, C. R. (1995b). Patient autonomy and the politics of professional relationships. *Journal of Advanced Nursing, 21*(1), 83–87.

May, C. R., & Fleming, C. (1997). The professional imagination: Narrative and the symbolic boundaries between medicine and nursing. *Journal of Advanced Nursing, 25*(5), 1094–1100.

May, C. R., & Purkis, M. E. (1995). The configuration of nurse–patient relationships: A critical view. *Scholarly Inquiry for Nursing Practice, 9*(4), 283–295.

McEwen, M., & Wills, E. M. (2007). *Theoretical basis for nursing* (2nd ed.). Lippincott Williams & Wilkins.

McKenna, H. (1997). *Nursing theories and models*. Taylor & Francis.

McKenna, H., & Slevin, O. (2011). *Vital notes for nurses: Nursing models, theories and practice*. John Wiley & Sons.

McNamara, M. S. (2010). Lost in transition? A discursive analysis of academic nursing in Ireland. *Nursing Science Quarterly, 23*(3), 249–256.

Meleis, A. I. (2007). *Theoretical nursing: Development and progress* (4th ed.). Lippincott Williams & Wilkins.

Meleis, A. I. (2012). *Theoretical nursing: Development and progress* (5th ed.). Wolters Kluwer/Lippincott Williams & Wilkins.

Mitchell, G. J., & Cody, W. K. (1992). Nursing knowledge and human science: Ontological and epistemological considerations. *Nursing Science Quarterly, 5*, 54–61.

Mitchell, G. J., & Cody, W. K. (2002). Ambiguous opportunity: Toiling for truth of nursing art and science. *Nursing Science Quarterly, 15*, 71–79.

Murphy, F., & Smith, C. (2013). *Nursing theories and models* (Three-volume set). Sage Publications.

Nelson, S. (1995). Humanism in nursing: The emergence of the light. *Nursing Inquiry, 2*(1), 36–43.

Nelson, S. (2000). *A genealogy of care of the sick: Nursing, holism and pious practice.* Nursing Praxis International.

Nelson, S. (2003). A history of small things. In J. Latimer (Ed.), *Advanced qualitative research for nursing* (pp. 211–230). Blackwell Science Ltd.

Nelson, S., & Gordon, S. (2004). The rhetoric of rupture: Nursing as a practice with a history? *Nursing Outlook, 52*(5), 255–261.

Newman, M. A. (1992). Prevailing paradigms in nursing. *Nursing Outlook, 40*(1), 10–32.

Newman, M. A., Sime, A. M., & Corcoran-Perry, S. A. (1991). The focus of the discipline of nursing. *Advances in Nursing Science, 14*(1), 1–6.

Paley, J. (2002). Caring as a slave morality: Nietzschean themes in nursing. *Journal of Advanced Nursing, 40*(1), 25–35.

Paley, J. (2006). Book review: Nursing theorists and their work. *Nursing Philosophy, 7*(4), 275–280.

Parker, J. M. (2004a). Theoretical perspectives in nursing: From microphysics to hermeneutics. In C. Taines (Ed.), *A body of work: Collected writings on nursing* (pp. 186–196). Nursing Praxis International. (Original work published 1988)

Parker, J. M. (2004b). Nursing on the medical ward. *Nursing Inquiry, 11*(4), 210–217.

Parse, R. R. (Ed.). (1987). *Nursing science: Major paradigms, theories, and critiques.* W. B. Saunders.

Parse, R. R. (1996). The human becoming theory: Challenges in practice and research. *Nursing Science Quarterly, 9,* 55–60.

Parse, R. R. (1997). The language of nursing knowledge: Saying what we mean. In I. M. King & J. Fawcett (Eds.), *The language of nursing theory and metatheory* (pp. 63–67). Sigma Theta Tau Monograph.

Petrovskaya, O. (2014a). Is there nursing phenomenology after Paley? Essay on rigorous reading. *Nursing Philosophy, 15*(1), 60–71.

Petrovskaya, O. (2014b). Domesticating Paley: How we misread Paley (and phenomenology). *Nursing Philosophy, 15*(1), 72–75.

Petrovskaya, O., Purkis, M. E., & Bjornsdottir, K. (2019). Revisiting "Intelligent nursing": Olga Petrovskaya in conversation with Mary Ellen Purkis and Kristin Bjornsdottir. *Nursing Philosophy, 20*(3), e12259.

Polifroni, E. C., & Welch, M. (Eds.). (1999). *Perspectives on philosophy of science in nursing: An historical and contemporary anthology.* Lippincott Williams & Wilkins.

Purkis, M., & Bjornsdottir, K. (2006). Intelligent nursing: Accounting for knowledge as action in practice. *Nursing Philosophy, 7*(4), 247–256.

Reed, P. G., & Shearer, N. B. C. (2009). *Perspectives on nursing theory* (5th ed.). Wolters Kluwer/Lippincott Williams & Wilkins.

Risjord, M. (2010). *Nursing knowledge: Science, practice, and philosophy.* Wiley-Blackwell.

Rodgers, B. L. (2005). *Developing nursing knowledge: Philosophical traditions and influences.* Lippincott Williams & Wilkins.

Rodriguez, R. T. (2011). Intelligible/unintelligible: A two-pronged proposition for queer studies. *American Literary History, 23*(1), 174–180.

Roy, C. (1988). An explication of the philosophical assumptions of the Roy adaptation model. *Nursing Science Quarterly, 1*(1), 26–34.

Roy, C., & Andrews, H. A. (1999). *The Roy adaptation model* (2nd ed.). Appleton & Lange.

Rudge, T. (1998). Skin as cover: The discursive effects of "covering" metaphors on wound care practices. *Nursing Inquiry, 5*(4), 228–237.

Sandelowski, M. (1993). Theory unmasked: The uses and guises of theory in qualitative research. *Research in Nursing and Health, 16*(3), 213–218.

Sandelowski, M. (2008). Reading, writing and systematic review. *Journal of Advanced Nursing, 64*(1), 104–110.

Sandelowski, M. (2011). When a cigar is not just a cigar: Alternative takes on data and data analysis. *Research in Nursing and Health, 34*(4), 342–352.

Thompson, J. L., Allen, D. G., & Rodriguez-Fisher, L. (Eds.). (1992). *Critique, resistance, and action: Working papers in the politics of nursing.* NLN.

Tomey, A. M., & Alligood, M. R. (Eds.). (2006). *Nursing theorists and their work* (6th ed.). Mosby.

Traynor, M. (1996). Looking at discourse in a literature review of nursing texts. *Journal of Advanced Nursing, 23*(6), 1155–1161.

Walker, L. O., & Avant, K. C. (2011). *Strategies for theory construction in nursing* (5th ed.). Pearson Prentice Hall.

White, J. (1995). Patterns of knowing: Review, critique, and update. *Advances in Nursing Science, 17*(4), 73–86.

Wilson, H. (2001). Power and partnership: A critical analysis of the surveillance discourses of child health nurses. *Journal of Advanced Nursing, 36*(2), 294–301.

2 Establishing the Field of Study

Postmodern, Post-structural, and Foucauldian Nursing Scholarship

In this chapter, I set the stage for further discussion by explaining my use of terminology, contextualizing postmodern and post-structural nursing scholarship, and describing my strategies for assembling the material for analysis. This preparation will help the reader to apprehend the contours of the postmodern, post-structural, and Foucauldian nursing field: the site for my research.

I begin by identifying the most noticeable continental philosophical influences on Anglophone nursing scholarship. After briefly addressing phenomenology and German critical theory, I arrive at postmodern and post-structural theory – the focus of my study. I discuss what I call "classification troubles." By this phrase, I mean that carving up the nursing intellectual community and literature according to labels such as "philosophy," "theory," "qualitative research"; "nursing" theory and "borrowed" theory; or even "postmodernism" as clearly separated from "post-structuralism" is counterproductive to an effort to understand the scope of postmodern/post-structural/Foucauldian nursing scholarship. Specifically, when nursing scholarship informed by the writings of French intellectual Michel Foucault is categorized in any one of these ways (e.g. in nursing curricula), this conception limits the visibility of post-structural writings and their potential to critically engage some foundational nursing discourses.

I then comment on the affinity of nursing scholarship to continental philosophical ideas that lend themselves to humanist and moralistic representations of nursing practice. For example, Habermas's normative ideas about communicative action capable of reducing power imbalances among participants in a conversation and Levinas's "ethic of the other" have been readily enlisted in nursing literature to support a holistic, caring, and person-centred account of the nurse–patient interaction. In contrast, post-structural ideas stemming from the stance of theoretical anti-humanism (e.g. de-centring the subject; turning attention from the subjects of the patient and the nurse to discourses structuring their subjectivities; and considering a capillary operation of power) complicate accepted accounts of nursing as benevolent caring. Because of the pervasive humanistic influences in nursing theory, both continental post-structural work and its rigorous applications in nursing run the risk of being misunderstood or dismissed in our discipline.

DOI: 10.4324/9781003194439-2

The object of my study was neither confined to strictly philosophical nursing literature nor literature clearly labelled as *post-structural,* which necessitated a broad scope for my analysis. The search strategies I employed[1] brought into view the contours of a sizable postmodern and post-structural nursing field, where Foucault was cited most frequently. Even a quick perusal of this vast literature reveals a remarkable difference in nursing scholarship informed by Foucault's ideas – the difference between American nursing theory literature and mostly non-American literature (i.e. British, Australian, and Canadian) originating outside of the canon of American nursing theory.

Continental Philosophy in Nursing: A Very Brief Overview

Continental philosophy is a broad intellectual tradition originating in continental Europe (e.g. Critchley, 2001; Sherrat, 2006; West, 2010). Standard introductions to continental philosophy mention its difference from analytic or Anglo-American philosophy (although some authors disagree about the usefulness of maintaining this contrast) and classify the most important directions of continental thought. These directions, in a roughly chronological order of appearance and arising as sets of responses to the ideas of earlier philosophers, most commonly include phenomenology, existentialism, critical theory, structuralism, postmodernism, and post-structuralism (e.g. Critchley, 2001, p. 13).

Continental philosophy, particularly when contrasted with analytic philosophy, can be usefully understood as "rooted in the historical, textual and theoretical modes of analysis" (Sherratt, 2006, p. 10). Rather than revolving around universal concepts that are ahistorical, continental philosophy is attentive to historical context. Continental styles of analysis are sensitive to linguistic tropes and expression. Further, continental philosophy values its beginnings in Greek, Roman, and Christian traditions, keeping this canon in play (Sherratt, 2006) even when undoing its foundations. Moreover, continental philosophical tradition has distinct intellectual concerns. For example, continental philosophy of social science perceives its object of inquiry, society, as "meaningful, often linguistic and historical" (Sherratt, 2006, p. 11). Where does meaning reside? How is meaning created and transmitted? "How is society historical?" (Sherratt, 2006, p. 12) are some of the central questions for continental philosophers.

Nursing literature reflects nurses' interest in the work of several continental philosophers. In the 1960s, nurse authors started to suggest that existentialist philosophy was relevant to nursing practice (Riemen, 1986, p. 87). Writings from the 1970s drew on phenomenological themes, such as existential intersubjective relating (Paterson & Zderad, 1976) and existential advocacy (Gadow, 1980). However, it was in the early 1980s that a kind of phenomenology most familiar to nurse researchers today – conceived of as a *research methodology* – was born.

From the 1980s, writings of German philosophers Edmund Husserl, Martin Heidegger, and Hans-Georg Gadamer and French phenomenologist Maurice Merleau-Ponty were increasingly transformed into a qualitative research methodology, nursing phenomenology and its varieties (e.g. Benner, 1985; Koch, 1995; Munhall & Oiler, 1986; Oiler, 1982; Omery, 1983; Parse et al., 1985). Phenomenology as a nursing qualitative methodology aimed to reveal subjective human experiences by means of lengthy, unstructured interviews. This approach gained a wide appeal among many nurse researchers. The importance of understanding patients' lived experiences and the meanings patients attribute to their illnesses has become nursing's unique goal, presented as transcending the narrow focus of biomedicine. Nursing phenomenological studies helpfully tap into how patients experience and understand their illnesses. More controversial, however, have been nurse phenomenologists' claims to adhere to continental philosophical phenomenology (see criticisms by Paley, 1997, 1998, 2000, 2005; Petrovskaya, 2014a, 2014b) and the early attempts by some authors (e.g. Munhall, 1982) to impose a "phenomenological paradigm" as nursing's exclusive approach to inquiry over the methods of "traditional science."

Around the mid-1980s, Frankfurt critical theory, primarily the works of philosopher Jürgen Habermas, generated an interest among American (e.g. David Allen, 1985, 1987; Allen et al., 1986; Hiraki, 1992; Ray, 1992; Thompson, 1985, 1987), Australian (e.g. C. Holmes & Warelow, 1997; Street, 1992), and Scandinavian (Holter, 1988) nurse scholars.[2] Habermas's ideas injected a fresh critical perspective into nursing science, as the following examples show. David Allen (1985) proposed critical-theoretical scholarship as a valuable form of nursing science complementing already established empirical-analytic and phenomenological-hermeneutic varieties of nursing science. Thompson (1987) connected nurses' recent interest in critical scholarship (Habermasian and feminist) to the growing contradictions in contemporary social and historical contexts, contradictions noticeable in the everyday working lives of many people: a close proximity of different ethnic groups and social classes, the corporate health care industry, and "white middle-class privilege" (p. 30). Thompson advocated for a critique of domination in nursing, that is, of "institutionalized power relations" (p. 27) anchored in gender, race, and class. She invited nurse scholars to bring these discussions into the classroom.

With the crucial assumption that language mediates social reality, Hiraki (1992) critiqued selected introductory nursing textbooks that depicted nursing practice in a limiting way: as a standardized, technical, and "scientific problem-solving approach" called *nursing process* (p. 1). She argued that nursing textbooks emphasized the instrumental rationality of nursing coupled with nurses' altruistic values. The textbooks, in Hiraki's analysis, contributed to significant problems: marginalization of the life-world of patients, denial of patients' agency, a lack of attention to practical issues related to communication between nurses and patients (such as conflict of values), and a decontextualized depiction of practice that proscribed the critique of institutional relations such as hospital policies.

In a non-American context, a nurse and sociologist from Ireland, Porter (1994), has reaffirmed the rational, value-based, emancipatory potential of Habermasian ideas for nursing practice by opposing them to what he described as relativism and an inadequate concept of power espoused by postmodern theory (Porter, 1996, 1997).

Considered against the background of a widespread acceptance by nurse scholars (particularly in North America) of the late Frankfurt School of thought, the problematization of Habermas's ideas is rare in nursing literature. Nelson (2000, p. x) and Nelson and Purkis (2004) argue that Habermas's theory of communicative action underpins the reflective practice designed by professional regulatory bodies in the United Kingdom and Canada as a mandatory mechanism to ensure nurses' continuing competence. These authors point out two problematic shifts disguised by the rhetoric of mandatory reflection: One is a shift of responsibility for nurses' ongoing skill development from the industry to individual providers. The other is a shift in focus from nurses' clinical performance to their ability to narratively account for their actions and thoughts: "Canadian nursing regulatory authorities have chosen to view competence as the rehearsal of ethical attributes consonant with the professional role, as opposed to the enactment of skilled conduct" (Nelson & Purkis, 2004, p. 247). These authors question the extent to which a reflection can be used as a proxy for nurses' competence.

I have been discussing how in the 1980s and early 1990s nurse scholars began to work with continental philosophical traditions of phenomenology and critical theory. Now, I turn to more recent continental philosophical traditions, postmodernism and post-structuralism. Because nursing *applications* of postmodernism and post-structuralism are the object of my argument, here I sketch only some of the key ideas commonly associated with these philosophical movements. Selected nursing literature presents credible – although dispersed – expositions of aspects of postmodern and post-structural theories and Foucault's and other philosophers' concepts (e.g. Aranda, 2006, pp. 136–137; Ceci, 2003; Cheek & Porter, 1997; Drummond, 2000 [on Nietzsche], 2001 [on Lyotard], 2002 [on Deleuze]; Fahy, 1997, pp. 27–28; A. Henderson, 1994; Porter, 1998; Springer, 2012; Thompson, 2007; Traynor, 2013).[3] Thus, the following synopsis is a glimpse into some of the key concepts and topics that can be usefully drawn upon in nursing and that have guided many nursing analyses.

As an intellectual movement, post-structuralism originated in the post- World War II France. Some of the most important theorists are Michel Foucault, Jacques Derrida, Gilles Deleuze, and Jean-François Lyotard. Notable French feminist post-structuralists are Julia Kristeva, Hélène Cixous, and Luce Irigaray. Post-structuralism influenced several academic fields across the world, most notably literary, social, and political theory. Post-structuralism was a reaction against Ferdinand de Saussure's linguistics and Claude Lévi-Strauss's anthropology, the two influential *structuralist* theories that grounded the understandings of language and culture on invariant structures. Post-structuralism is characterized by a stance of theoretical anti-humanism – a de-centring of the human subject. In contrast to the transcendental phenomenological subject, the human subject in post-structural theory is viewed not as the author of her "experiences" but as the product of discourses (i.e. not as an originator of discourses but as their effect). Thus, post-structuralism posits the primacy of language in the construction of human reality. Discourses systematically create the objects of which they speak. However, discourses are not separate from material realities; they include institutional practices and produce material effects. According to Foucault, discourses operate within the power/knowledge nexus: Power is understood as regimes of truth coextensive with the kinds of knowledges that it makes possible. Foucault conceptualizes power as capillary, existing conterminously with resistances, and productive of desires and objects. This view contrasts with the earlier and highly prevalent conceptions of power: power as contaminating otherwise "power-free" genuine relationships or knowledge; power as held and wielded in a society by a few "powerful" ones at the top of the social hierarchy; and power as suppressing and saying "no."

Postmodernism is characterized by a suspicion towards the metanarratives of progress based on Reason;[4] of the autonomous, free, and rational individual; and of the grand emancipatory projects promising freedom from oppression. In other words, postmodernism rejects the assumptions of modernism – humanism and a progressive view of history. Postmodernism posits a challenge to essences (e.g. essential identities) and signals the emergence of the politics of difference. It invites the deconstruction of binary thinking. Postmodernism celebrates the "death of the Author" and the turn to intertextuality, or recognition that authorial intent (the psychology of the individual writer) cannot fix the meaning of the text, which always "cites" other texts and is thus open to multiple interpretations. Clearly, theoretical anti-humanism and incredulity towards the metanarratives of progress and emancipation – the key postmodern and post-structural ideas – hold the potential to unravel many of nursing's conceptions. Throughout the book I examine how this did or did not happen.

A useful starting place to establish the contours of a postmodern and post-structural nursing field is to appreciate the circuits of its production and circulation. When did the first references to these philosophical movements and central theorists appear in nursing literature? What are the key scholarly groups and individual nurse authors applying postmodern and post-structural theory? What kinds of scholarly writing fall within the categories of postmodern and post-structural work? Of the French theorists, who is cited most? How does postmodern and post-structural scholarship fit within the larger continentally informed nursing field? I address these crucial questions in the following and throughout the book.

In nursing, the first citations of the work of the French philosopher and social theorist Michel Foucault appeared in the late 1980s, two of them in the British *Journal of Advanced Nursing*.[5] In the earliest article citing Foucault, Lees and co-authors (1987) unmask the quality assurance (QA) programs introduced across health care settings in the United Kingdom as motivated by the considerations of systems efficiency and the attempts to safeguard professional interests. The authors argue that the demand for standardization inherent in QA promotes a "nursing gaze" (e.g. the breaking down of patients' issues and lives into small components) analogous to a medical gaze critiqued by Foucault. Another British nurse author, Chapman (1988), utilized Foucault's notions of power and discipline to analyse the enactment of the nursing professional therapeutic discourse in ward reports. In 1989, in the American journal *Advances in Nursing Science*, Dzurec (1989) turned to Foucault's conception of power/knowledge to pursue a different aim – to reconcile the American nursing academic debates about the legitimacy of a phenomenological paradigm versus a traditional, "positivist" paradigm in nursing science. Subsequently, from the early 1990s onwards, on both sides of the Atlantic and in Australia, nurse scholars have increasingly embraced French postmodern and post-structural thought. Intriguingly, this interest manifested in quantitatively and qualitatively asymmetric ways between American and non-American nursing literature. My study surfaces and probes this asymmetry.

Classification Troubles: Postmodern vs. Post-Structural . . . Philosophy vs. Theory

Referring to continental philosophy of the latter half of the 20th century, I use the terms *philosophy* and *theory* interchangeably. This usage reflects labelling vagaries characteristic of 20th-century continental thought. First, some thinkers like Hannah Arendt steadfastly rejected identification as a philosopher (Stack Altoids, 2013). Others, like Foucault or Derrida, are said to express ambivalence about categories of structuralism versus post-structuralism, or indeed, any categories. Second, the multidisciplinary educational backgrounds of the prominent figures of the French intellectual scene (e.g. history and social science for Foucault, literary criticism for Barthes) confound classification efforts. Finally, an interdisciplinary existence – perhaps a forced exile – of continental theory to the departments of literary criticism, political science, sociology, or cultural studies, specifically, in North America (Cusset, 2008), further complicates the drawing of a clear division between philosophy and theory.

It is worth noting that nursing literature informed by postmodern and post-structural writings does not attempt to pin them down as either philosophy or theory; indeed, such attempts would contradict postmodernism's emphasis on blurring boundaries and inverting hierarchies. However, although American metatheoretical and methodological nursing literature displays a range of uses of the terms *philosophy* and *theory* (e.g. Sandelowski, 1993), influential classifications of nursing knowledge have imposed preferred and lasting connotations to these notions. For example, Fawcett's (2005) "structure of nursing knowledge" rigidly defines and distinguishes between philosophy, conceptual models, and theory. Moreover, as my next chapter explains, within this structure, "nursing theory" is valorized while the status of "borrowed theory" (i.e. theories from other disciplines) is precarious. I argue in this book that the American disciplinary matrix of "unique nursing knowledge" (more accurately, its variations), although toying with Foucault's ideas, produces highly selective visibility and intelligibility for nursing scholarship informed by postmodern and post-structural theory.

Similarly, it is unproductive to try to separate relevant nursing scholarship into either postmodernist or post-structuralist camps. A quick survey of nursing journals publishing continentally informed work reveals that this distinction is rarely drawn by the authors, and when it is, this step does not imply some principled distinction, but is rather a matter of echoing the sources one uses. Commonly, bibliographies in nursing articles and books are composed of multiple sources that a reader conversant with contemporary cultural and social theory can identify as originating from sociology, anthropology, literary criticism, or philosophy, and exemplifying postmodern and post-structural theory alongside other kinds of critical theory. Within the same publications, we encounter references to Foucault's work alongside the work of the following social scientists, philosophers, and theorists: Goffman (Davies & Davina Allen, 2007; Martin Johnson & Webb, 1995); Kristeva (Rudge, 1998); Haraway (Rudge, 1999); J. Butler (Crowe, 2000); Latour (Purkis, 2001); and Derrida, Barthes, Lyotard, and Rorty (Rolfe, 2000; Stevenson & Beech, 2001).

In some respect, blurred boundaries between the two "isms" seem acceptable not only to nurses but to scholars in the humanities. For example, short introductions to postmodernism (C. Butler, 2002) and post-structuralism (Belsey, 2002) – with their otherwise specific contents – both address Althusser's notion of ideology, Barthes's "death of the Author," Derrida's deconstruction, Foucault's discourse, Lyotard's grand narratives, and Saussure's linguistics. Moreover, these two books refer to Freud, Marx, and Lévi-Strauss, as well as the notions of text, power, and truth. The overlap between the two movements is evident, and rather than attempting to fully separate them, the authors in nursing and other disciplines focus on what is most important: how postmodernism and post-structuralism depart from and challenge ideas and practices – both intellectual and material practices – that preceded them in the West. In other words, the attention is on how these "post"(s) opened up new understandings and different practices in spheres of human life as diverse and interconnected as politics, culture, arts, literature, theory, ethics, science, education, and health.

Although humanities literature that focuses on continental philosophy usually differentiates between postmodern and post-structural theory, these distinctions rarely enter nursing literature. Nurses commonly draw on a mix of "postmodern" writers, Foucault being chief among those. For this reason, I use the terms *post-modern theory* and *post-structural theory* nearly interchangeably throughout the book, unless the subject under discussion demands a clear separation.

A general trend in the United States was to refer to theory exported from France from the late 1960s onwards as French theory (Cusset, 2008). If the type of blurring invoked above accompanies a sympathetic reception of postmodern and post-structural ideas, there is also a rather unsympathetic view that impatiently labels "all these ideas" as "postmodernist jargon." In the hands of detractors of French theory, the word "postmodernism" became an all-encompassing and derogatory name. In nursing, we hear echoes of this annoyance with the "postmodernist hoax" in Clarke (1996), Glazer (2001), and Garrett (2018, Chapter 5).[6]

One further caveat about identifying and categorizing postmodern and post-structural nursing work relates to a common and often correct assumption that this body of publications exemplifies nursing *philosophical* scholarship. Emanating from a broad continental tradition, these philosophical movements indeed do find themselves at home in journals like *Nursing Philosophy* or *Nursing Ethics* and among scholarly groups like the International Philosophy of Nursing Society (IPONS). But this grouping based on *philosophy* kinship will offer us only a limited view into postmodern and post-structural theorizing in nursing. For example, a review of the first decade of IPONS membership revealed that only a few nurse members, who self-identified as nurse-philosophers, have explicitly positioned their work in the continental stream (most notably, John Drummond and Gary Rolfe); some other IPONS members have been trained as philosophers in the analytic tradition (e.g. Stephen Edwards; John Paley, and Mark Risjord). But the latter authors, too, find selective continental ideas useful. In other words, French-inspired philosophical scholarship in nursing is not limited to members of philosophical groups.

In fact, a vast majority of nurse authors writing in a postmodern or post-structural vein do not self-identify as *nurse-philosophers*. Notably, some of the influential continentally informed authors in nursing have a background in the social sciences and humanities: David Allen in theatre history and philosophical phenomenology; Joanna Latimer and Sam Porter in sociology; Carl May in economics; Sioban Nelson in history; Judith Parker in psychoanalysis; Trudy Rudge in anthropology; and Michael Traynor in literary studies/English literature.

These authors often forgo typical descriptors like "nursing philosophy" or "qualitative research," but their continentally based analyses or critiques do not suffer from this ostensible lack of classification. Further, another small group of Foucauldian nurse scholars, called *In Sickness and In Health*, spearheaded and continues to organize conferences that are emphatically interdisciplinary, engaging scholars from nursing, allied health disciplines, the humanities, and the social sciences. In nursing, unsurprisingly, we often witness productive dialogue and collaboration among continentally based philosophizing and selected sociological approaches (e.g. Dorothy Smith's institutional ethnography, Harold Garfinkel's ethnomethodology, and Bruno Latour's actor-network theory). To recap, in the previous discussion, I aimed to complicate accepted positioning of nursing postmodern and post-structural theorizing as either "nursing philosophy" or "qualitative research" by pointing out many directions in which this theorizing has entered our discipline and evolved.

French Theory and Nursing: Uncomfortable Bedfellows?

At a glance, in the discipline of nursing, humanistic and normative strands of continental philosophy enjoy wider recognition and easier acceptance than antihumanist, "relativistic" postmodern and post-structural theory as well as other continental analyses not easily transformable into a moral rulebook. The ethical propositions of French phenomenologist Emmanuel Levinas (see Nortvedt, 1998, 2001, 2003, as one particularly strong supporter) and a communicative rationality outlined by Habermas (e.g. Hiraki, 1992; Holter, 1988; Mill et al., 2001; Porter, 1994; Ray, 1992; Sarvimaki, 1988; Sumner, 2001) have never met any doubt or resistance on ethical grounds.[7] In contrast, "postmodernism" and Foucault's work generated a marked reaction against their moral ambiguity (Francis, 2000; Kermode & Brown, 1996; Porter, 1996, 1997) and suggestions to remedy their perceived shortcomings (e.g. Falk Rafael, 1997; Reed, 1995; Watson, 1995). These attitudes amount to a censorship of "borrowed" ideas to ensure their "fit" with nursing's values. Such a preference for a particular kind of theory/philosophy can be traced historically in the American nursing theoretical discourse, as the following section demonstrates.

Early Use of the Term Philosophy in American Nursing Science

As early as 1952, authors in the *Nursing Research* journal expressed concerns over rapidly shifting nurses' roles (Risjord, 2010, p. 13). Nurse leaders worried about clinical nurses' gradual move away from direct patient care to managerial roles and an increasing interference with care by burgeoning technologies. Nurses found particularly troubling that these changes were prompted by social factors beyond nurses' reflective and intentional action (Risjord, 2010, p. 14). Academic leaders envisioned the following solution to this situation: The nursing discipline would formulate a philosophy of nursing that clarifies what nursing practice should be and expresses its essential values. A question *What is nursing?* has become, from the 1960s, an ideological disciplinary anchorage; *the* question for the discipline. In the words of Risjord (2010), the "call for a philosophy of nursing was thus a call to define nursing, to find its heart, and thereby defend a nurse's proper role" (p. 13). Thus, from the mid-20th century, for many academic nurse leaders, the question *What is nursing?* presupposed a philosophical – not an empirical – answer.

Concerns about the erosion of nursing clinical practice resonate as acutely today as they did in the 1950s. Perhaps this historical example reflects a fundamental continuity in the conception of the relation between the nursing discipline and practice and helps us understand the role of "a philosophy/theory of nursing" in mediating this relationship. Nursing practice, today more than in the past, follows the logic of a capitalist market economy whose interests are removed from an ideal altruistic vision of nursing. This is the context for a certain sense of anxiety or urgency that accompanies the disciplinary call to return to "the foundational question," *What is nursing?* and to write "new nursing philosophies/nursing theories," that is, to firmly stake a claim about what nursing practice should look like and to counter the problematic realities of practice. Such a conception of a nursing philosophy – as an aspirational statement, an ideal vision, and a values manifesto – has been shaping the attitudes towards continental philosophy/theory in nursing discourse.

Influential American theoretical nursing literature (Chinn, 1997; Mitchell & Cody, 1992; Watson, 2005, pp. xiii, 3) tends to conceive of a theory/philosophy (of and for nursing) as depicting "what should be" rather than "what is": "ideal" rather than "real." This preference for futuristic and hope-imbued theory partially explains an unrecognized attitude towards philosophies/theories that enter nursing from other disciplines. As long as a "borrowed" theory lends itself to an extraction of morals, it is accepted and assimilated. Think of the widely popular but often simplified notions of phenomenology and critical social theory that have been adopted within philosophy statements in some nursing departments. The curricular translations of such philosophies draw student attention to patients' lived experiences and client empowerment and emancipation. Student nurses are enticed to judiciously use power that their position confers and to "share" it with their patients. Those nurse authors who go further and specify their appeal to critical theory often cite Habermas. This late Frankfurt critical theory enjoys a good reputation in nursing; its normative character likely explains its popularity.

The difficulty with other strands of continental theory, on the other hand, is that they are neither normative nor prescriptive. Often, these strands unpack "what is" without reassuring the reader about a preferred future. Although continental thought is clearly value-laden, its values, rather than being humanistic (human-centred; positing human consciousness as the originator of language and meaning), often advocate theoretical anti-humanism. In analyses of nursing practices, the latter stance invites unpacking nurses' actions and words rather than accepting them at face value. In most illustrative cases, continental theorists doubt human altruistic motives (Friedrich Nietzsche), the extent of the subject's agency (Foucault), one's ability to account for one's self (Judith Butler), and the fruitfulness of emancipatory action (Jacques Lacan). I have witnessed the strain with which nursing audiences met Paley's (2002) critique of holistic, caring, phenomenological nursing philosophy that he brusquely equated, à la Nietzsche, to the *ressentiment* of slaves (nursing) revolting against the higher values of nobles (medicine). Embracing post-structural thought, we deal with a paradox: Continental theory, being critical, propels us to think, yet the outcome of thinking is "dangerous," not predetermined. Critical theory (in a broad sense) defies drawing moralistic conclusions.

Thinking "infected" by continental ideas may well unravel nurses' cherished ideologies. Such was the explosive effect of nurses' discovery of Foucault: Nurses, far from being downtrodden as the literature often portrays them, are in fact powerful agents of the state carrying out its biopolitical agenda (D. Holmes & Gastaldo, 2002). The pursuit of post-structural questioning can lead us into the heart of present-day nursing foundations: Considering post-Enlightenment critiques of rationality and the autonomous subject, what is the fate of nursing's conception of the autonomous nurse and patient (Drevdahl, 1999; see also Ceci, 2012)? Or, what are the implications of Foucault's and J. Butler's problematization of subjectivity and account-ability for nurses' mandatory practice of producing self-reflective narratives as a learning and professional development tool (Nelson & McGillion, 2004; Nelson & Purkis, 2004)? If seriously considered, these questions invite a revision of many core nursing ideals/ideas, especially the pervasive humanistic assumptions of American nursing theory (Mulholland, 1995; Nelson, 1995; Traynor, 2009).

For critics, postmodern and post-structural French philosophy outrageously lacks explicit moral, altruistic commands (Soper, 1986, Chapters 6 and 7) and smacks of being an "uncomfortable bedfellow" for nursing (Francis, 2000). Reservations towards French theory in nursing literature can be placed in the context of this unease. Further, conceiving philosophy (of and for nursing) as an ideal(ized) vision or as a moral compass cannot accommodate anti-humanist and materialist philosophies that confound human agency by positing the co-constituting role of power, discourse, the subconscious, historical contingency, or economic conditions in/on nursing practice. Clearly, the analytic relevance of French theory for understanding aspects of nursing practice can be recognized more fully when a narrow conception of a "proper disciplinary theory/philosophy" is challenged.

Time Frame for Book's Analysis

Since the late 1980s, when references to Foucault first appeared in nursing journals, more than a thousand articles, book chapters, and books employed (as a primary or complementary theoretical tool) postmodern, post-structural, and/ or Foucault's ideas to discuss or analyse diverse topics in nursing knowledge, research, and practice. In this book, I zoom in on the first two decades of this scholarly literature to most effectively convey the contrast between different streams within this literature. Why have I chosen this particular time frame?

First, according to my bibliometric analysis (see note 1 in this chapter), the period from 2005 to 2009 appears to be the heyday for nursing post-structural/ Foucauldian scholarship, based on the record number of articles in the leading journals: *Journal of Advanced Nursing* (*JAN*), *Nursing Inquiry* (*NI*), and *Nursing Philosophy* (*NP*). Around 2010, some journals that actively published post-structural and Foucault-informed scholarship (i.e. *Advances in Nursing Science* [*ANS*] in the United States and *JAN* in the United Kingdom) have noticeably shifted their attention towards other priorities (see Chapter 5, note 5, and Chapter 6, note 3).

Second, I made two intriguing observations about nursing postmodern/post-structural/Foucauldian scholarship, in 2008 and 2012 respectively: observations that called for the exploration of events spanning the 1990s to the early 2010s. In 2008, Sioban Nelson, editor of *NI*, participated in the panel discussion at a conference for the Canadian Association for the History of Nursing in Toronto. She commented on nurse academics' rising interest in Foucault's ideas and invited the audience to move from quantity to quality in their scholarship when developing manuscripts citing Foucault.

Not long after this, in the fifth edition of the compendium on American nursing theory, Afaf Meleis (2012) asserted that postmodernism and post-structuralism were not useful to nursing. Specifically, she claimed that postmodernism was not relevant in the field of medical sociology, and therefore "similar assumptions could be made about its utility for nursing science" (p. 149). The contrast was striking: an American nurse theorist dismissing postmodernism and post-structuralism versus an Australian-Canadian nurse scholar, who spearheaded the leading Foucauldian nursing journal, *NI*, describing significant interest in Foucault's work in nursing. What happened from the late 1980s to the 2010s that resulted in this asymmetry? I look closely at this period to investigate.

My analysis presents a counterpoint to commentaries in nursing literature that crudely equated, wholesale, so-called postmodern and French-inspired nursing scholarship with charlatanism. The first two decades of Foucauldian nursing scholarship especially strongly reveal the hues in various nurses' application of postmodernism and post-structuralism, thus demonstrating that it is foolish to outrightly reject any nursing discourse appealing to French theory.

The reader will notice that the Appendix includes occasional sources beyond 2010. When I had these sources readily available, rather than removing them for the sake of preserving the neat cut-off point, I opted to include them as further illustration of patterns described in the book.

Concluding Thoughts

Nurses in the academy have long used continental philosophical works to inform their writings. The humanistic and emancipatory orientations of phenomenology, German critical theory, and second-wave feminism easily align with nursing's ideals. Other traditions of continental philosophy, postmodernism and post-structuralism, were rejected by some as non-normative and relativist. However, from the late 1980s and into the 21st century, a vast field of postmodern and post-structural nursing scholarship has developed. The French philosopher most influential in nursing is Michel Foucault. While first citations to his work appeared almost simultaneously in the British *Journal of Advanced Nursing* (JAN) and American *Advances in Nursing Science* (ANS) in the late 1980s, Foucauldian scholarship differed widely in American nursing theoretical literature and outside of this canon. The three non-American nursing journals – JAN, *Nursing Inquiry*, and *Nursing Philosophy* – have led in publishing a significant volume of post-structural scholarship, mostly by Australian, British, and Canadian nurses. In contrast, the leading U.S. journal ANS contains a much smaller set of papers informed by post-structural ideas, predominantly by American authors. My book aims to explore this asymmetry. In addition, many post-structural articles in U.S. nursing literature seem to indicate specific concerns unique to the American nursing intellectual scene. To understand these concerns, I turn to the following chapter to discuss conceptions of theory and science in the discipline of nursing in the United States, or what I call the American intellectual disciplinary matrix.

Notes

1 For my analysis in the book, I relied on extensive electronic library searches to retrieve articles from Anglophone nursing journals in addition to manual and snowball literature searches (e.g. for books) based on my familiarity with relevant scholarly networks. In 2015, I searched the *Web of Science* and the Cumulative Index to Nursing and Allied Health Literature (CINAHL) databases, using library-recommended variations of keywords *post-structuralism* and *Foucault*. I manually screened all results to weed out irrelevant records and estimate the scope of postmodern, post-structural, and

Foucauldian nursing scholarship from the late 1980s to the early 2010s. In the following text, I present the most significant search results.

Using the keyword "post-structuralism" in CINAHL resulted in 295 relevant papers: 70 in the *Journal of Advanced Nursing* (*JAN*) established in 1976; 96 in *Nursing Inquiry* (*NI*) established in 1994; 33 in *Nursing Philosophy* (*NP*) established in 2000; 20 in *Advances in Nursing Science* (*ANS*) established in 1978; 11 in *Nurse Researcher* (*NR*); 12 in the *Journal of Psychiatric and Mental Health Nursing* (*JPMHN*); 7 in the *Journal of Clinical Nursing* (*JCN*); 4 in *Nursing Ethics* (*NE*); and a smaller number in several other journals. *Aporia*, a Canadian online nursing journal launched in 2009 at the University of Ottawa, was likely not indexed in CINAHL in 2015. In this list, only one journal, *ANS*, represents an overt interest in American nursing theory.

Selected comparisons:

- From 1989 to 1999, *NI*, although launched only in 1994, published the highest number of papers (19), followed by *JAN* (15) and *ANS* (5).
- From 2000 to 2004, *NI* (27) and *JAN* (24) led again, while *ANS* and the new journal *NP* published 13 and 14 papers, respectively. In other journals, like *NR* and *JPMHN*, the term *post-structuralism* started appearing in the early 2000s.
- The years 2005 to 2009 were a heyday for scholarship employing post-structural ideas. In total, 94 articles were published, 10 more than during the previous five years and almost twice as many as from 1989 to 1999. In the period from 2005 to 2009, *NI* (25), *JAN* (22), and *NP* (14) maintained the level of the previous five years, while *ANS*'s numbers dropped markedly (from 13 to 2). Over the same period, *NR*, *JPMHN*, *JCN*, and *NE* published a few papers each, an increase over previous years.
- A significant change occurred during 2010–2015. The overall number dropped to 69, with the most noticeable reduction occurring in *JAN* (9 which is less than half of the previous level) and *NP* (5 which is one-third of the previous level). No papers mentioning post-structuralism appeared in *ANS*. In contrast, *JCN* (5), *NR* (4), and especially *JPMHN* (8) demonstrated an increased number of references to post-structuralism. As before, however, *NI* led and maintained the record number of 25 articles.

Needless to say, these numeric comparisons make no claim about the quality of post-structural nursing scholarship.

This comparison of the volume of post-structural papers in English from 1989 to 2015 demonstrates a tenfold difference between the three leading non-American journals (*JAN*, *NI*, *NP*) and the leading American journal, *ANS*. To determine how many American nurse scholars were publishing in the top three (from the previous list) non-American journals, I checked authors' addresses and found that only 10 per cent of post-structural papers in *JAN*, *NI*, and *NP* (17 of 199) were by American authors. In turn, only 10 per cent (2 of 20) post-structural papers in *ANS* were by non-Americans. Indeed, the majority of publications in *JAN*, *NI*, and *NP* were authored by nurses from Australia, the United Kingdom, and Canada. Similarly, Gastaldo and D. Holmes (1999) noted a preponderance of Australian nursing publications informed by Foucault, which were mostly published in *JAN* and *NI*. Traynor (2006), in his analysis of discourse-analytic studies published in *JAN* from 1996 to 2004, reported that of the 24 reviewed papers, 15 were from the United Kingdom or Ireland, 7 from Australasia, and 1 from the United States.

In a separate search, I used the keyword *Foucault* (in All Text) in CINAHL. Nurse scholars whose work is informed by post-structural ideas do not always employ the terms *postmodernism* or *post-structuralism* but rather cite thinkers commonly identified with these overlapping philosophical movements. Thus, my previous search, while resulting in a large volume of relevant journal articles, might have screened out important examples of nursing work (e.g. sociological analyses, nursing history) that theorize nursing practices in a post-structural vein without ever applying the shorthand labels for philosophical movements. Examples are the first two applications of Foucault's work presented in *JAN* by British authors Lees et al. (1987) and Chapman (1988). These articles were not identified through the previous search because the authors do not describe their analyses informed by Foucault as post-structural.

After an initial screening, I estimated that approximately 750 papers are relevant. From 1987 to December 2015, most references to Foucault appeared in the following nursing journals published in English: *JAN* (211), *NI* (170), *NP* (77), *JCN* (76), *JPMHN* (60), *NE* (27), *NR* (19), and *ANS* (18). Articles retrieved in the two searches (295 and 750) overlapped significantly, yet the Foucault-informed set usefully expanded and supplemented the post-structural set.

The American postmodern, post-structural, and Foucauldian nursing field – comprised of journal papers (Table A1 in the Appendix) and references in nursing textbooks (Table A2) – is relatively modest. Thus, I attempted to create a comprehensive picture by bringing together all those American sources I found. In contrast, non-American Foucauldian scholarship is more voluminous. However, it is possible to identify central scholarly groups, conferences, and individuals contributing to that vast field. Thus, I focused on the books and book chapters authored or edited by nurse academics who cite Foucault (Table A3). Some of these authors are known for their long-standing and productive interest in Foucault's work. Others cite Foucault in a minor way, while drawing on other social theory and philosophy. Still other nurse authors criticize Foucault's ideas. As expected, nurses who published or edited books have also actively contributed to journal publications retrieved through my searches. The basis for selection will become apparent throughout the chapters devoted to American and non-American Foucauldian scholarship.

What I do not address within the scope of my book are interdisciplinary allied health journals or Anglophone nursing journals from Brazil and Scandinavia. Finally, nursing studies citing Foucault are too numerous for my current work as I am interested in painting on a large canvas. Nursing studies citing Foucault, for example, encompass several nursing discourse-analytic studies, which have been perceptively analysed and critiqued (Buus, 2005; Traynor, 2006), so when relevant, I draw on these criticisms.

To my knowledge, this ambitious work of bringing together the postmodern, post-structural, and Foucauldian nursing field and distinguishing its American nursing theory and non-American varieties is the first attempt in nursing.

2 Since the 1990s, many nurse scholars have found useful the work of various critical philosophers – those representing the early and late Frankfurt school as well as Paulo Freire. Here I refer to only some of the influential, pioneering nursing publications.

3 A peculiar characteristic of some nursing writings that claim to draw on continental philosophy – in this case, postmodern and post-structural theory – is a disconnect between often good expositions of philosophical precepts and subsequent analyses that contradict these precepts. (For this reason, I opted to indicate specific page numbers for some articles.) I have written about this issue in relation to phenomenological nursing research (Petrovskaya, 2014a).

4 *Reason*, or *Enlightenment rationality*, refers to a belief that humankind is "becoming progressively self-directed in thought and action through the awakening of one's intellectual powers, lead[ing] ultimately to a better, more fulfilled human existence" (Bristow, 2017).

5 To reiterate a point I made earlier, *JAN* is designated as a British journal based on its continuous tradition of a British editorship and on its high record of publishing postmodern and post-structural articles written by British authors.

6 Two other articles, Francis (2000) and Kermode and Brown (1996), while also critical of postmodernism and its relevance to nursing, are more nuanced and offer interesting ideas to consider. For example, Kermode and Brown draw on selected authors in the humanities like Fredric Jameson who rejected postmodernism as the cultural logic of late capitalism, inadequate to grapple with the real political and economic oppressions of a capitalist society.

7 One exception is Edwards's (2014) scepticism about the necessity of an additional layer of reality, "moral realism," as proposed by Nortvedt.

References

Allen, D. G. (1985). Nursing research and social control: Alternate models of science that emphasize understanding and emancipation. *Image: The Journal of Nursing Scholarship, 17*(2), 58–64.

Allen, D. G. (1987). The social policy statement: A reappraisal. *Advances in Nursing Science, 10*(1), 39–48.

Allen, D. G., Benner, P., & Diekelmann, N. (1986). Three paradigms for nursing research. In P. Chinn (Ed.), *Nursing research methodology: Issues & implementation* (pp. 23–28). Aspen Publishers.

Aranda, K. (2006). Postmodern feminist perspectives and nursing research: A passionately interested form of inquiry. *Nursing Inquiry, 13*(2), 135–143.

Belsey, C. (2002). *Poststructuralism: A very short introduction*. Oxford University Press.

Benner, P. (1985). Quality of life: A phenomenological perspective on explanation, prediction, and understanding of nursing science. *Advances in Nursing Science, 8*, 1–14.

Bristow, W. (2017). Enlightenment. In E. N. Zalta (Ed.), *The Stanford encyclopedia of philosophy*. https://plato.stanford.edu/archives/fall2017/entries/enlightenment/

Butler, C. (2002). *Postmodernism: A very short introduction*. Oxford University Press.

Buus, N. (2005). Nursing scholars appropriating new methods: The use of discourse analysis in scholarly nursing journals 1996–2003. *Nursing Inquiry, 12*(1), 27–33.

Ceci, C. (2003). Midnight reckonings: On a question of knowledge and nursing. *Nursing Philosophy, 4*(1), 61–76.

Ceci, C. (2012). "To work out what works best": What is good care in home care. In C. Ceci, M. E. Purkis, & K. Björnsdóttir (Eds.), *Perspectives on care at home for older people* (pp. 81–100). Routledge.

Chapman, G. (1988). Reporting therapeutic discourse in a therapeutic community. *Journal of Advanced Nursing, 13*(2), 255–264.

Cheek, J., & Porter, S. (1997). Reviewing Foucault: Possibilities and problems for nursing and health care. *Nursing Inquiry, 4*(2), 108–119.

Chinn, P. L. (1997). Response to "Ethics and the geography of the nurse–patient relationship." *Scholarly Inquiry for Nursing Practice, 11*(1), 61–63.

Clarke, L. (1996). The last post? Defending nursing against the postmodernist maze. *Journal of Psychiatric & Mental Health Nursing, 3*(4), 257–265.

Critchley, S. (2001). *Continental philosophy: A very short introduction*. Oxford University Press.

Crowe, M. (2000). The nurse–patient relationship: A consideration of its discursive context. *Journal of Advanced Nursing, 31*(4), 962–967.

Cusset, F. (2008). *French theory: How Foucault, Derrida, Deleuze, & Co. transformed the intellectual life of the United States* (J. Fort, Trans.). University of Minnesota Press.

Davies, B., & Allen, D. (2007). Integrating "mental illness" and "motherhood": The positive use of surveillance by health professionals. *International Journal of Nursing Studies, 44*(3), 365–376.

Drevdahl, D. (1999). Sailing beyond: Nursing theory and the person. *Advances in Nursing Science, 21*(4), 1–13.

Drummond, J. S. (2000). Nietzsche for nurses: Caring for the Ubermensch. *Nursing Philosophy, 1*, 147–157.

Drummond, J. S. (2001). Petits différends: A reflection on aspects of Lyotard's philosophy for quality of care. *Nursing Philosophy, 2*(3), 224–234.

Drummond, J. S. (2002). Freedom to roam: A Deleuzian overture for the concept of care in nursing. *Nursing Philosophy, 3*(3), 222–233.

Dzurec, L. (1989). The necessity for and evolution of multiple paradigms for nursing research: A poststructuralist perspective. *Advances in Nursing Science, 11*(4), 69–77.

Edwards, S. D. (2014). Moral realism in nursing. *Nursing Philosophy, 15*(2), 81–88.

Fahy, K. (1997). Postmodern feminist emancipatory research: Is it an oxymoron? *Nursing Inquiry, 4*(1), 27–33.

Falk Rafael, A. R. (1997). Advocacy oral history: A research methodology for social activism in nursing. *Advances in Nursing Science, 20*(2), 32–44.

Fawcett, J. (2005). *Contemporary nursing knowledge: Analysis and evaluation of nursing models and theories* (2nd ed.). F. A. Davis.

Francis, B. (2000). Poststructuralism and nursing: Uncomfortable bedfellows? *Nursing Inquiry, 7*(1), 20–28.

Gadow, S. (1980). Existential advocacy: Philosophical foundation of nursing. In S. Spicker & S. Gadow (Eds.), *Nursing: Images and ideals. Opening dialogue with the humanities* (pp. 79–101). Springer Publishing Company.

Garrett, B. (2018). *Empirical nursing: The art of evidence-based care.* Emerald Publishing Limited.

Gastaldo, D., & Holmes, D. (1999). Foucault and nursing: A history of the present. *Nursing Inquiry, 6*(4), 231–240.

Glazer, S. (2001). Therapeutic touch and postmodernism in nursing. *Nursing Philosophy, 2*(3), 196–212.

Henderson, A. (1994). Power and knowledge in nursing practice: The contribution of Foucault. *Journal of Advanced Nursing, 20*(5), 935–939.

Hiraki, A. (1992). Tradition, rationality, and power in introductory nursing textbooks: A critical hermeneutics study. *Advances in Nursing Science, 14*(3), 1–12.

Holmes, C. A., & Warelow, P. J. (1997). Culture, needs and nursing: A critical theory approach. *Journal of Advanced Nursing, 25*(3), 463–470.

Holmes, D., & Gastaldo, D. (2002). Nursing as means of governmentality. *Journal of Advanced Nursing, 38*(6), 557–565.

Holter, I. (1988). Critical theory: A foundation for the development of nursing theories. *Scholarly Inquiry for Nursing Practice, 2*(3), 223–236.

Johnson, M., & Webb, C. (1995). Rediscovering unpopular patients: The concept of social judgement. *Journal of Advanced Nursing, 21*(3), 466–475.

Kermode, S., & Brown, C. (1996). The postmodernist hoax and its effects on nursing. *International Journal of Nursing Studies, 33*(4), 375–384.

Koch, T. (1995). Interpretive approaches in nursing research: The influence of Husserl and Heidegger. *Journal of Advanced Nursing, 21*(5), 827–836.

Lees, G., Richman, J., Salauroo, M., & Warden, S. (1987). Quality assurance: Is it professional insurance? *Journal of Advanced Nursing, 12*(6), 719–727.

Meleis, A. I. (2012). *Theoretical nursing: Development and progress* (5th ed.). Wolters Kluwer/Lippincott Williams & Wilkins.

Mill, J. E., Allen, M. N., & Morrow, R. A. (2001). Critical theory: Critical methodology to disciplinary foundations in nursing. *Canadian Journal of Nursing Research, 33*(2), 109–127.

Mitchell, G. J., & Cody, W. K. (1992). Nursing knowledge and human science: Ontological and epistemological considerations. *Nursing Science Quarterly, 5*, 54–61.

Mulholland, J. (1995). Nursing, humanism and transcultural theory: The "bracketing-out" of reality. *Journal of Advanced Nursing, 22*(3), 442–449.

Munhall, P. L. (1982). Nursing philosophy and nursing research: In apposition or opposition? *Nursing Research, 31*(3), 176–177, 181.

Munhall, P. L., & Oiler, C. J. (Eds.). (1986). *Nursing research: A qualitative perspective.* Appleton-Century-Crofts.

Nelson, S. (1995). Humanism in nursing: The emergence of the light. *Nursing Inquiry, 2*(1), 36–43.

Nelson, S. (2000). *A genealogy of care of the sick: Nursing, holism and pious practice.* Nursing Praxis International.

Nelson, S., & McGillion, M. (2004). Expertise or performance? Questioning the rhetoric of contemporary narrative use in nursing. *Journal of Advanced Nursing, 47*(6), 631–638.

Nelson, S., & Purkis, M. E. (2004). Mandatory reflection: The Canadian reconstitution of the competent nurse. *Nursing Inquiry, 11*(4), 247–257.

Nortvedt, P. (1998). Sensitive judgement: An inquiry into the foundations of nursing ethics. *Nursing Ethics, 5*(5), 385–392.

Nortvedt, P. (2001). Needs, closeness and responsibilities: An inquiry into some rival moral considerations in nursing care. *Nursing Philosophy, 2*(2), 112–121.

Nortvedt, P. (2003). Subjectivity and vulnerability: Reflections on the foundation of ethical sensibility. *Nursing Philosophy, 4*(3), 222–230.

Oiler, C. (1982). The phenomenological approach in nursing research. *Nursing Research, 31,* 178–181.

Omery, A. (1983). Phenomenology: A method for nursing research. *Advances in Nursing Science, 5*(2), 49–63.

Paley, J. (1997). Husserl, phenomenology and nursing. *Journal of Advanced Nursing, 26*(1), 187–193.

Paley, J. (1998). Misinterpretive phenomenology: Heidegger, ontology and nursing research. *Journal of Advanced Nursing, 27*(4), 817–824.

Paley, J. (2000). Against meaning. *Nursing Philosophy, 1*(2), 109–120.

Paley, J. (2002). Caring as a slave morality: Nietzschean themes in nursing. *Journal of Advanced Nursing, 40*(1), 25–35.

Paley, J. (2005). Phenomenology as rhetoric. *Nursing Inquiry, 12*(2), 106–116.

Parse, R. R., Coyne, A. B., & Smith, M. J. (Eds.). (1985). *Nursing research: Qualitative methods.* Brady Communications.

Paterson, J., & Zderad, L. (1976). *Humanistic nursing.* Wiley & Sons.

Petrovskaya, O. (2014a). Is there nursing phenomenology after Paley? Essay on rigorous reading. *Nursing Philosophy, 15*(1), 60–71.

Petrovskaya, O. (2014b). Domesticating Paley: How we misread Paley (and phenomenology). *Nursing Philosophy, 15*(1), 72–75.

Porter, S. (1994). New nursing: The road to freedom? *Journal of Advanced Nursing, 20*(2), 269–274.

Porter, S. (1996). Contra-Foucault: Soldiers, nurses and power. *Sociology, 30*(1), 59–78.

Porter, S. (1997). The patient and power: Sociological perspectives on the consequences of holistic care. *Health & Social Care in the Community, 5*(1), 17–20.

Porter, S. (1998). *Social theory and nursing practice.* Macmillan Education UK.

Purkis, M. (2001). Managing home nursing care: Visibility, accountability and exclusion. *Nursing Inquiry, 8*(3), 141–150.

Ray, M. A. (1992). Critical theory as a framework to enhance nursing science. *Nursing Science Quarterly, 5*(3), 98–101.

Reed, P. (1995). A treatise on nursing knowledge development for the 21st century: Beyond postmodernism. *Advances in Nursing Science, 17*(3), 70–84.

Riemen, D. J. (1986). The essential structure of a caring interaction: Doing phenomenology. In P. L. Munhall & C. J. Oiler (Eds.), *Nursing research: A qualitative perspective* (pp. 85–108). Appleton-Century-Crofts.

Risjord, M. (2010). *Nursing knowledge: Science, practice, and philosophy.* Wiley-Blackwell.

Rolfe, G. (2000). *Research, truth, and authority: Postmodern perspectives on nursing.* Macmillan Press.

Rudge, T. (1998). Skin as cover: The discursive effects of "covering" metaphors on wound care practices. *Nursing Inquiry, 5*(4), 228–237.

Rudge, T. (1999). Situating wound management: Technoscience, dressings and "other" skins. *Nursing Inquiry, 6*(3), 167–177.

Sandelowski, M. (1993). Theory unmasked: The uses and guises of theory in qualitative research. *Research in Nursing and Health, 16*(3), 213–218.

Sarvimaki, A. (1988). Nursing care as a moral, practical, communicative and creative activity. *Journal of Advanced Nursing, 13*(4), 462–467.

Sherratt, Y. (2006). *Continental philosophy of social science: Hermeneutics, genealogy, and critical theory from Greece to the twenty-first century.* Cambridge University Press.

Soper, K. (1986). *Humanism and anti-humanism.* Hutchinson.

Springer, R. A. (2012). Michel Foucault: A man of a thousand paths, a thousand faces, and a thousand emerging relevancies. *Aporia, 4*(1), 51–56.

Stack Altoids. (2013, April 8). *Hannah Arendt "Zur Person" full interview (with English subtitles).* [Video file] (Original interview conducted in 1964). https://youtu.be/dsoImQfVsO4

Stevenson, C., & Beech, I. (2001). Paradigms lost, paradigms regained: Defending nursing against a single reading of postmodernism. *Nursing Philosophy, 2*(2), 143–150.

Street, A. F. (1992). *Inside nursing: A critical ethnography of clinical nursing practice.* State University of New York Press.

Sumner, J. (2001). Caring in nursing: A different interpretation. *Journal of Advanced Nursing, 35*(6), 926–932.

Thompson, J. L. (1985). Practical discourse in nursing: Going beyond empiricism and historicism. *Advances in Nursing Science, 7*(4), 59–71.

Thompson, J. L. (1987). Critical scholarship: The critique of domination in nursing. *Advances in Nursing Science, 10*(1), 27–38.

Thompson, J. L. (2007). Poststructuralist feminist analysis in nursing. In Sr. C. Roy & D. A. Jones (Eds.), *Nursing knowledge development and clinical practice* (pp. 129–144). Springer Publishing Company.

Traynor, M. (2006). Discourse analysis: Theoretical and historical overview and review of papers in the *Journal of Advanced Nursing* 1996–2004. *Journal of Advanced Nursing, 54*(1), 62–72.

Traynor, M. (2009). Humanism and its critiques in nursing research literature. *Journal of Advanced Nursing, 65*(7), 1560–1567.

Traynor, M. (2013). Discourse analysis. In C. T. Beck (Ed.), *The Routledge international handbook of qualitative nursing research* (pp. 282–294). Routledge.

Watson, J. (1995). Postmodernism and knowledge development in nursing. *Nursing Science Quarterly, 8*(2), 60–64.

Watson, J. (2005). *Caring science as sacred science.* F. A. Davis.

West, D. (2010). *Continental philosophy: An introduction* (2nd ed.). Polity Press.

3 American Nursing Science and Discipline-Specific Theory

In the Grips of Logical Positivism

In the second half of the 20th century, a logical positivist model of science exerted a subterranean influence on the development of the nursing discipline. In this chapter, I summarize a systematic critique of this influence undertaken by Mark Risjord (2010) and thus provide a background to the founding ideas of American nursing science. Over decades and across theoretical literature, these ideas coalesced into what I refer as the historically produced intellectual frame of reference in the discipline of nursing, or a *matrix of intelligibility*. A "consensus view of the 1970s" (Risjord, 2010) in American scholarly nursing literature posited that scientific disciplines develop a unique, discipline-specific set of theories; theories necessarily include abstract and general laws; and the testing of a theory presupposes the deduction of hypotheses from the laws (a deductive-nomological, pyramid-like logical structure of theory). Two decades into the 21st century, much of American theoretical discourse displays these beliefs. Moreover, it is not decisive for the endurance of these ideas that they are whole-heartedly held or universally shared in the discipline of nursing; what matters is a constant circulation of vocabulary/literary tropes and of practices of "knowledge development" stemming from logical-positivist conceptions and indicative of certain conventions in a scholarly community. It appears that nursing writings and genres adhering to one or another version of this intellectual matrix (and that operate with particular formal terminology, i.e. grand theory, middle-range theory, practice-level theory, borrowed theory, metaparadigm, paradigms, or models of knowledge development based on "patterns of knowing") have been granted the "nursing knowledge" status, making other conceptions of theory as well as practices of theorizing unintelligible forms of nursing knowledge. I argue that this intellectual matrix has powerfully shaped the reception and evolution of postmodern and post-structural thought in American nursing theoretical writings in the 1990s and into the 2000s. After outlining the significance of Risjord's work for my analysis, I turn to examine the scene of American nursing science drawing on Risjord's ideas.

Significance of Risjord's Work

In this section, I explain why Risjord's critiques warrant centre stage in this chapter, what the boundaries of his analysis are, and how I use his argument as a

DOI: 10.4324/9781003194439-3

springboard to develop my perspective. Mark Risjord, a philosopher of science at Emory University in the United States, taught graduate nursing courses on knowledge development for nearly a decade (Risjord, 2010, p. xiii) before publishing a systematic analysis of knowledge development in nursing.[1]

What makes Risjord's (2010) analysis worthy of an in-depth exploration? Although explicit critiques of logical positivism or "positivism" appeared in nursing literature as early as the 1970s and nurse authors since have claimed a distance from this philosophy of science (e.g. David Allen, 1985; Chinn, 1985; Dzurec, 1989; Gortner, 1993/1997; Munhall, 1982; Reed, 1995; Rodgers, 2005; Silva & Rothbart, 1984/1997; Watson, 1995), the following discussion demonstrates the typical inconsistency between such claims and actual metatheoretical formulations in nursing literature. Risjord's decisive examination detailed the full degree and depth of influence that logical positivism exerted on American nursing theory. For example, critique of logical positivism in nursing has taken the following forms: Webster et al. (1981) rejected views of theories as being true or false, science as value free, and the scientific method as the only valid method of inquiry. Meleis (1997) listed the following characteristics of the received view of science contested by nurses: objectivity, deduction, one truth, and generalization. In contrast to these representations of logical positivism, Risjord (2010) argued first that some of these characteristics are not bound to logical positivism and do not have negative implications assigned to them in nursing literature. And second, most important, Risjord argued that other features of logical positivism permeate nursing literature yet remain unnoticed.

There are specific boundaries to Risjord's analysis that determine the points of my departure beyond his work. He focuses on the domain of "nursing science,"[2] namely, on the *theoretical* discourses explicitly identified as "*science*," to the exclusion of other practices of theorizing in American nursing literature (such as theorizing found in the analyses of empirical findings or discussions of various topics, e.g. in Liaschenko [1994, 1997; Liaschenko & Fisher, 1999; Liaschenko & Peter, 2004], Sandelowski [1999, 2000], or Drevdahl [1999], who do not position their work as "science"). Further, Risjord elucidates only *analytic-philosophical* influences on nursing, that is, he does not trace the sociological roots – also strong – of nurses' conceptions of theory. Finally, his analysis presents a composite, robust version of the pyramid conception of American nursing science and theory, whereas individual nursing writings operate with *elements* of that conception, often articulating divergent points of view on "nursing knowledge." Therefore, I examine how *non-scientific* – postmodern and post-structural – philosophical ideas were received and shaped within the dominant intellectual matrix of American nursing theory. Further, tracing selected sociological influences assists in comparing American and non-American nursing works. I am also interested in teasing apart specific postmodernism-sensitive discursive positions within the broader American nursing knowledge terrain. These three intellectual pursuits take Risjord's apt argument as a starting point. Drawing on his analysis, I will now present an understanding of science and theory that grounds American nursing theory's vision of a unique nursing discipline.

The Formation of Nursing Science

The second half of the 20th century is ubiquitously acknowledged in American nursing history as a period of intensive development in nursing education and research. The decades from the 1950s to 1980s are perceived as an impressive move forward for nursing as a discipline and a profession. The image of a desirable profession that motivated nurses was worked out based on the analyses of established professions like medicine in the early 20th century and later reiterated in sociological literature. This image included, among its crucial attributes, a unique body of knowledge (e.g. Dingwall, 1975; Hughes, 1963; Larsen & Baumgart, 1992; Ross Kerr, 1996). As Risjord (2010) retrospectively summarizes, "The drive to create a nursing profession was, perhaps, the most important motive for the rise of nursing research" (p. 8). A path to professionalize the vocation of nursing would necessarily entail creating the nursing *discipline* as both a field of post-secondary study *and* a unique body of knowledge taught in those programs.

In his synthesis of theories about professions, sociologist Andrew Abbott (1988) found that professions usually have some special *abstract* skill that sets them apart from other groups (p. 7). A profession – in this case nursing – exerts control through controlling a system of abstract knowledge: "[P]ractical skill grows out of an abstract system of knowledge, and control of the occupation lies in control of the abstractions that generate the practical techniques" (p. 8). Furthermore, Abbott distinguished nursing as a "subordinate jurisdiction" to the profession of medicine, requiring constant maintenance of that subordination. It seems inevitable, then, that American nurse theorists would be actuated to build a system of abstract theories that announced their status as a profession while also functioning to contest and resist nursing's subordination to medicine.

Several factors supported the growth of academic nursing in the latter part of the 20th century. The U.S. government began funding nursing research focused on the nursing workforce in the late 1940s (Risjord, 2010, p. 11). In 1952, the journal *Nursing Research* was established. An increasing number of nurses were pursuing graduate studies. In the 1960s, nurses commonly earned doctoral degrees in education and biomedical sciences. This was followed by a professional aspiration, in the 1970s and early 1980s, to educate future academics in nursing from a "nursing perspective" (Grace, 1978; Rodgers, 2005, p. 5; see also Gortner, 1991, and Newman, 1972). These developments depended upon and further fuelled the idea of establishing nursing research and building the knowledge base of nursing.

In some academic nursing departments in the United States, the project of building "the knowledge base specific to nursing" was firmly conceptualized, early in the process, as *nursing science* and, moreover, has adhered to a particular model of science. Some nurse scholars envisioned nursing as a *basic* science – similar to other sciences in the academy – with its own conceptual apparatus, laws, and subject matter (Risjord, 2010, p. 82). A logical positivist model of science that underpinned this vision dominated the mid-20th-century broader academic landscape. At that time, the main tenets of logical positivism, known in the philosophy of science as "the received view of theory," were widely influential across the natural and social sciences. Adoption – knowingly or otherwise – of the received view by nurse scholars, set the direction for the discipline: "To be a discipline, . . . nursing needed unique theories at a high level of abstraction. These were unified into a basic science by shared concepts and themes (the meta-paradigm)" (Risjord, 2010, p. 5).

Historically, logical positivism has not always grounded nursing science. A careful look at early nursing publications allows one to distinguish a shift in thinking about science and theory (Risjord, 2010). In the 1950s, when the notion of nursing science started appearing in the literature, it usually referred to the natural and social sciences that had traditionally supported nursing practice, namely, biological, psychological, and social (Risjord, 2010, p. 12). Nurse leaders like Virginia Henderson called for clinical nursing research based on these sciences. Related to this, when nurse authors referred to theory, they meant "a systematic consolidation of natural and social scientific findings relevant to nursing practice" (Risjord, 2010, p. 12).

From 1930 to 1960, the majority of research related to nursing was conducted by non-nurses at the request of governmental agencies and focused on human resource management and requirement for and cost of services (Gortner, 2000, p. 61). Even in the early years of *Nursing Research*, "studies of the nurse" published in this journal greatly outnumbered "studies of nursing practice" (V. Henderson, 1956, as cited in Gortner, 2000, p. 61). In the early 1960s, federal grants promoted the latter kind of research: studies of "effects of performance of nursing acts on the patient. . .; effects on nursing of changing patterns of nursing care and changing health needs, and nursing in different illness categories" (Gortner, 2000, p. 61). A retrospective look confirms that since that time these various types of clinical, behavioural, outcome, and evaluation research have been carried out in the discipline (Gortner, 2000, p. 64; Risjord, 2011). From a point of view of nurse academics conducting these studies, a collective body of this research constituted nursing science. A bifurcation in American nursing emerged in the 1960s and 1970s: on the one hand, a minority group of nurse theorists interested in metatheoretical issues and debating philosophy of nursing science, including prescriptions for research flowing from or contributing to unique nursing theories, and on the other hand, a majority of nurse researchers whose practices relied on theories from various other disciplines (see also Risjord, 2011). Moreover, it appears that the taken-for-granted designation of "nursing science" as denoting nursing research has shifted, or has been monopolized, to mean the activities and intellectual output of the former group, American nurse theorists (Diers, 1994; see also other chapters in McCloskey & Grace, 1994). The following discussion in this chapter concerns metatheoretical scholarship generated mostly by the authors collectively identified as nurse theorists, philosophers, and metatheoreticians.

Throughout the 1960s in American nursing literature, although the idea became widespread that nursing is a scientific discipline in its own right that presupposes theoretical activity, the nature of this activity was debatable. Nurse scholars argued about the relationship between the discipline (i.e. research, theory) and clinical practice as well as the character of nursing theory (Risjord, 2010, p. 20). Several authors (Conant, 1967; Dickoff & James, 1968; Ellis, 1969) independently articulated a set of perspectives that can be summarized as "practice theory," following Florence Wald and Robert Leonard (1964), professors of nursing and sociology, respectively, from the Yale University School of Nursing. In this view, clinical practice guides research and theory; the discipline is expected to solve problems in practice. Nursing knowledge is "specialized" to the discipline of nursing – it is *nursing* knowledge – because it blends the knowledge from relevant other sciences to address *nursing* issues. Because of its close connection to practice, theoretical activity displays nursing values and goals (Risjord, 2010, p. 21). However, this conception of nursing science was soon to become a minority view.

The change occurred in the 1970s, when, in Risjord's (2010) words, a "consensus" took place about the way nursing knowledge and the academic discipline of nursing were to be conceived. Although opinions of individual scholars might have varied, the agreement (captured in the most influential publications of the 1970s onwards) held that nursing is a unique science with the distinctive, hierarchical disciplinary structure and a corresponding, multi-level picture of theory. According to Risjord (2010), and as became easier to discern in retrospect, this consensus has followed, often uncritically and without full awareness, the assumptions of logical positivist science.[3] But what is logical positivism? What specific view of science and theory does this philosophical position entail? In what ways has this received view of theory influenced nursing scholarship? And what might be the implications of this influence, within the discipline of nursing, towards alternative ways to theorize? I take a closer look at these questions in the remaining part of this chapter.

As will become evident, the long-lasting effects of the 1970s consensus on nursing *science* have been uncovered by authors whose work I cite, most notably Risjord (2010). The effects of a logical positivist view of theory on explicitly *non-scientific* nursing scholarship (primarily in the United States), however, have been eclipsed, partly due to a prevailing, and largely uncritical, conception of nursing as a science.[4] Yet, I argue in this study that modelling American nursing theory and the "unique discipline" upon a logical positivist conception of science also had consequences for how non-scientific intellectual currents – in this case, postmodern and post-structural continental thought – entered and evolved in nursing theoretical writings from the late 1980s through approximately the first decade of the 21st century – the period of interest for my study.

A Logical Positivist Conception of Theory

A Note on Terminology

Risjord (2010) began by clarifying key terminology widely used in nursing discussions on the philosophy of science. It must be noted that clarifying key terms according to philosophical conventions may still not illuminate their various uses in nursing literature and may even raise further questions, for example, about the suitability of the term "empiricism" with its commitment to empirical data to describe the largely speculative, non-observation-based strands of American nursing theory. These challenges aside, Risjord's analysis usefully exposes subterraneous philosophical assumptions of American nursing theory.

Logical positivism (or simply "positivism," or "logical empiricism") is "a particular way of working out the commitments of empiricism" (Risjord, 2010, p. 85). Empiricism is an epistemological position; in other words, it is not an ontological one in that it does not say what kinds of phenomena exist. As an epistemological position, empiricism claims that all knowledge arises from experience, that is, from observation (Markie, 2015, "Empiricism," para. 1). This view contrasts with rationalist epistemology that posits that knowledge is acquired solely from reasoning and reflection. Further, logical positivism presupposes a specific view of the structure of knowledge, namely, "forming successively more powerful generalizations out of the raw material of observation" (Risjord, 2010, p. 85). At the outset of the discussion of positivism it is also important to emphasize that "positivism" is not synonymous with "quantitative research," the negative connotation sometimes perpetuated in nursing literature erroneously seeking to deepen the rift between quantitative and qualitative research.

The Vienna Circle

Developed by the scholars of the Vienna Circle, logical positivism exerted maximum influence in the 1930s and 1940s and then gradually lost the support of philosophers in the late 1950s. The following synopsis provides some details about the Vienna Circle. Any synopsis carries a risk of grossly oversimplifying decades of dense arguments in the philosophy of science. Further, the Vienna group generated highly heterogeneous views on some important points, although with a sufficient overlap to allow me to talk about its doctrines (Uebel, 2014, "Introductory Remarks," paras. 3 and 4). The "received view of scientific theories," critiqued by Risjord (2010), came into prominence after World War II and was closely associated with (although not identical to) the Vienna Circle doctrines (Uebel, 2014, "Selected Doctrines and their Criticisms," para. 2).

The philosophers of the Vienna circle envisioned a unified science without a distinction between the natural and the social sciences (Uebel, 2014, "Overview of Doctrines," para. 4). In the early 20th century, this generated protest from German philosophers Wilhelm Dilthey and Edmund Husserl among others.

The Vienna Circle modelled their vision of philosophy on the knowledge claims of logic and mathematics, which "gained their justification on purely formal grounds, by proof of their derivability by stated rules from stated axioms and premises" (Uebel, 2014, "Overview of Doctrines," para. 2). The central doctrine of logical positivism is called the *verification principle*. It states that all significant propositions could be reduced to statements about sense experiences or observations. Thus, the meaning of a proposition is the method of its verification. Metaphysics are meaningless, as are any propositions that cannot be verified in a specified way. Logical positivism also rejected the knowledge claims of normative ethics (Uebel, 2014, "Overview of Doctrines," para. 3). Logical positivism demanded formalist analyses, that is, analyses "given solely in terms of the logical relations of these concepts and propositions to other concepts and propositions . . . us[ing] the tools of formal logic" (Uebel, 2014, "Verificationism and the Critique of Metaphysics," para. 10). Next, the logical positivism-inspired, received view of scientific theory posited a theory–observation dichotomy. Theoretical terms have meaning only insofar as they can be transformed, by logically devised bridge laws, to observational terms. The latter are interpreted, whereas the theoretical terms are not (Uebel, 2014, "Scientific Theories, Theoretical Terms and the Problem of Realism"). Finally, logical positivism viewed science as cumulative and ahistorical.

Various critiques in the philosophy of science pointed out the weaknesses of logical positivism. Logical positivism cannot account for phenomena such as electrons and black holes because they cannot be directly observed. Famously, Thomas Kuhn's argument about scientific revolutions offered a competing account of a history of science (Uebel, 2014, "The Vienna Circle and History," para. 2). Most relevant to my discussion are critiques pointing out the inability of the received view of scientific theory to account for actual scientific practices and theories. The logical positivist conception of theory, also called the *syntactic view* ("an axiomatized collection of sentences"), has been undermined by the semantic view (a theory is "a collection of non-linguistic models"), and both have been challenged by the pragmatic view (a theory is "an amorphous entity consisting perhaps of sentences and models, but just as importantly of exemplars, problems, standards, skills, practices and tendencies") (Savage, 1990, cited in Winther, 2015, "Introduction," para. 1). While a full correspondence between the tenets of logical positivism and American nursing theory cannot be claimed, further in the following I describe the received conception of theory as it has played out in nursing according to Risjord (2010).

Rejected by the Philosophers of Science, Unwittingly Embraced by Nurses

In fact, "as nurses were discovering and adopting. . . [the logical positivist, received view of theory], philosophers of science were abandoning it" (Risjord, 2010, p. 82). Risjord persuasively argues that the influence of logical positivism on nursing is so entrenched and subtle that its traces are still tangible even in writings of those nurses who explicitly reject this position. Indeed, in the foreword to Risjord's book, nursing professor Sue Donaldson confesses that she did not recognize a pervasive presence of logical positivism and was surprised by Risjord's findings (Donaldson, 2010, p. xvii).

To surface for the reader the unrecognized and deep presence of logical positivism, Risjord (2010) teases out three mechanisms of its influence. The most explicit demonstration of the impact is when nurse authors intentionally and directly advocated the logical positivist conception of science. This, however, has rarely occurred; on the contrary, nurses rhetorically distanced themselves from the pejoratively tinted "positivism," especially with the rise of postpositivist critiques in the philosophy of science. All the while, contradicting this rhetoric, nurse authors (e.g. Fawcett, 2005, pp. 4, 19, 23; B. Johnson & Webber, 2010; Newman, 1972, p. 84; L.O. Walker & Avant, 2011) approvingly cite chief philosophical defenders of the received view of theory like Carl Hempel, Ernest Nagel, and Herbert Feigl. Related ideas about theory construction came into nursing from certain American sociological texts of the 1960s–1970s. Although links between these ideas and logical positivism are not straightforward, the sociologists Jack Gibbs, Jerald Hage, and Jonathan Turner, cited in nursing literature (e.g. Fawcett, 2005; Hardy, 1978; L. O. Walker & Avant, 2011), advocated a particularly structured, formal theory. However, Gibbs (1994, p. 90) commented that formal theory construction in sociology was short-lived and fell out of favour in the 1970s.[5]

Ironically, as logical positivism was becoming outdated in philosophy and sociology, those nurse authors swayed by the logical positivist philosophy of science and by formal sociology gained authority in the discipline. Risjord (2010, p. 97) cautions that the logical positivist influence through citation, although it appears to mostly belong to the historical past, has produced another, philosophical, offshoot. Breathing the air of the positivist theoretical currents in the academy, nurse theorists developed their *own* ideas, that is, not directly traceable to any particular source but rather resembling those ideas "in the air." Consequently, while the straight adherents of logical positivism have had to grapple with the postpositivist criticisms (e.g. by Kuhn and Laudan), nurses' "own" scientific ideas often remained immune to those challenges.

What Is a Proper Science and a Proper Theory?

According to the logical positivist view, the hallmark of science is the creation and testing of theory:

> Scientific theory was supposed to have a particular logical structure: it was a set of abstract and general laws. By specifying values for the variables or other initial conditions, testable hypotheses could be deduced from theory. If the hypotheses conflicted with observation, the theories would have to be modified. Scientific research was thus a matter of theory development and testing.
>
> (Risjord, 2010, p. 16)

Some nurse scholars set their goal on science-like theory development. Many of them embraced the main tenets of logical positivism and the consequences of this position for understanding scientific disciplines. Risjord (2010, p. 95) teases out those beliefs: Scientific knowledge articulates the fundamental laws of (human) nature. These laws are expressed as axioms, or first principles, of a theory. Within the empiricist framework of logical positivism, scientific knowledge is possible because observational statements can be derived from laws and tested. Scientific theory should possess explanatory power, which means deducing explanations from the laws. Each scientific discipline, like physics, chemistry, and biology, is defined by its own set of theories with axioms and concepts unique to those disciplines. These are characteristics of a basic science.[6]

Further, nursing science accepted two cornerstone assumptions of logical positivism, namely value-freedom of scientific theory and a distinctive logical structure of scientific theory (Risjord, 2010, p. 22). Risjord comments that Lorraine Walker was one of the first nurse authors who clearly introduced these ideas in the early 1970s. L. O. Walker's (1971) argument for the value-freedom of scientific theory depended on her separation of the three domains – science, philosophy, and praxiology – each with an independent set of concerns. Philosophy is concerned with *what should be*, that is, the speculative ends of nursing practice; praxiology looks after the practical means of achieving those ends, for example, testing nursing interventions; whereas science is strictly about describing and explaining the current state of affairs. In other words, the value-positing domain of philosophy and the value-free domain of science do not overlap.

Another characteristic of scientific theory that L. O. Walker (1971) strongly advocated was its distinctive structure. In technical terms, this is a deductive-nomological structure or the received view of theory (Risjord, 2010, p. 23). Theory consists of several levels; each level of theory is supported by the level below it. Imagine a pyramid: At the top, theory begins with the most abstract general laws (*nomos*), from which less-abstract propositions are derived by a process of mathematical or logical deduction. Those propositions are tested by observation or experiment. If a low-level theory is disconfirmed, it threatens the levels above, necessitating revision of the higher-level theory. This hierarchical form of theory, upheld in logical positivist science and intimately familiar in nursing, is visually displayed, for example, in Newman (1972) and Fawcett (2005, pp. 4, 20). A pyramid helps us to visualize the model of science pervasive in nursing (Risjord, 2010).[7]

Logical Positivist Beliefs in Nursing Science

Definitions of Theory

Risjord (2010) observes that the writings of several noted nurse theorists (e.g. Abdellah, King, Newman, Roy, and D. Johnson) reveal profound influences of the logical positivist, value-free, deductive-nomological vision of science and theory (p. 23). Definitions of theory found in several nursing publications present the most telling examples, as can be seen in the following quotation:

> Concepts are connected in a theory by verbal or mathematical statements called propositions. Propositions describe the theoretical linkages between concepts. Two types of propositions are generally found in a theory. Axioms, or initial propositions, are the starting points for derivations; they are not to be tested, but rather taken as givens in the theory. In contrast, postulates,

also called deduced propositions or theorems, are statements of supposition regarding the type of relation between the concepts of the theory. A theory's explanatory power is found in its postulates.

(Fawcett, 1978/1997, p. 717)

Theory appears as a deductive-nomological structure. Risjord devotes a full page to similar quotations from four other authoritative, representative nursing articles from the 1970s. Noteworthy, when I was enrolled in an undergraduate "nursing knowledge" course in 2004, we learned a similar definition of theory. A view of theory, long rejected in the philosophy of science (e.g. Hacking, 1983; Laudan, 1984/1999; van Fraassen, 1980/1999a, 1980/1999b), still circulates in current editions on nursing disciplinary knowledge.

It might be warranted at this point to reiterate my earlier observation. Likely, the ideas about theory expressed in complicated definitions such as Fawcett's are neither strongly adhered to nor even well understood by the wider nursing audiences. The remarkable endurance of these ideas, however, depends on a constant circulation of this specialized vocabulary in a host of nursing theory guides and anthologies.

Value-Free or Value-Laden?

Risjord (2010) points out the following paradox: While nurse theorists favourably cite mid-20th-century scientific views and lay them as a ground for their own theorizing, these nurses' writings expose two incoherencies. First, nurse authors do not always recognize the logical positivist roots of their ideas. For instance, nurse theorists Hesook Suzie Kim and Callista Roy explicitly denied such influences (Gortner, 1993/1997). Second, despite positive references to scientific value-freedom, nurses' theoretical output is thoroughly (though appropriately for nursing) value-laden. The following quotation from Sue Donaldson and Dorothy Crowley (1978) illustrates the lack of value-neutrality in that the authors clearly prefer certain outcomes when they identify the subject of nursing inquiry as "concern with the principles and laws that govern the life processes, *well-being*, and *optimum* functioning of human beings – sick or well. . . . Concern with the processes by which *positive* changes in health status are affected" (Donaldson & Crowley, 1978, p. 113; italics added). The notions of *well-being*, *optimum functioning*, *positive changes*, and *health* are overtly judgemental; they presuppose clear value commitments (Risjord, 2010, pp. 62–63).

According to Risjord (2010, 2011), another example of a logical positivist-influenced view of science as a value-free endeavour is an erroneous separation of nursing science (empirics) from nursing values (ethics) and a concomitant separation of theoretical knowledge (i.e. discursively formulated empirical knowledge) from practical knowledge (i.e. "aesthetic and personal knowing" as non-discursive know-how) epitomized in Barbara Carper's (1978) hugely influential article "Fundamental Patterns of Knowing in Nursing." This recurrent and unwitting assertion of the value-freedom of science obfuscates moral and political commitments embedded in nursing (empirical) theoretical work (Risjord, 2010, 2011, p. 500; Yeo, 1989). Risjord (2010) urges that "nursing knowledge must be both normative and descriptive" (p. 55). He uses these examples to stress – against the assumption of value-freedom in logical positivist science – an acceptance of values within postpositivist philosophy and a constitutive role of values in nursing theory and research.

These examples of nursing writings also give rise to another question. How do we explain the following paradox? Nursing science literature declares a distance from "outdated positivism," while at the same time favourably citing this philosophy of science, yet in the next move produces writings that contradict the very ideas cited. It appears that the misunderstanding of philosophical ideas, or at least a highly selective reading, has historically accompanied nurses' engagement with the philosophy of science (Hussey, 2001; Kim & Kollak, 2006; Paley, 2006).

The Structure of Nursing Knowledge

In the foregoing sections, I cited a noted nurse scholar, Jacqueline Fawcett, professor of nursing at the University of Pennsylvania. From the late 1970s, throughout the 1980s and 1990s, and more recently, she has contributed a significant volume of metatheoretical work to the discipline of nursing, including her book, *Contemporary Nursing Knowledge: Analysis and Evaluation of Nursing Models and Theories* (2005). Fawcett's authoritative voice and the work of synthesizing and profiling the American nursing theoretical field are influential (see Slevin, 2003, pp. 161–162, on the influence of Fawcett's ideas in the United Kingdom). Arguably, Fawcett's work reflects the most robust version of the consensus view of theory. This understanding of theory and elements of the discipline constantly reinforces the idea of a unified and unique nursing knowledge cautious towards "borrowed theory." From the vantage point of my argument, namely surfacing the conditions of (un)intelligibility of postmodern and post-structural philosophy in nursing, Fawcett's legacy is problematic.

Fawcett (2005) developed the "structural holarchy of contemporary nursing knowledge" (p. 4). This structure orders all nursing knowledge according to the level of abstraction: the most abstract conceptual models on top, followed by grand theory, then middle-range theory, to concrete and specific empirical indicators on the bottom. The structure's crown, the four metaparadigm concepts (person, environment, nursing, and health), are said to circumscribe nursing's unique domain and to direct research in the discipline.

Returning to one of the previous points, we recall that "practice theorists" proposed the reverse direction for the discipline, starting *from* clinical practice. In the 1960s, two positions on the "discipline–practice" hierarchy were debated. Several prominent nurse scholars like Dorothy Johnson (1959) and Rozella May Schlotfeldt (1960) posited that the *discipline* of nursing would set the agenda for nursing research and theory development. The initial step in this process is a formulation of a philosophy of nursing, which defines the domain of nursing. Flowing from the philosophy, theories will be developed and tested. These theories will then become an intellectual basis of nursing clinical practice. As mentioned earlier, Wald and Leonard (1964), Dickoff and James (1968), and Ellis (1969) contested this view. They argued for "practice theory": Problems that arise in nursing practice will prompt research, whose outcome in the form of a theory will be tested and applied to solve those problems. Practice theory was called *situation-producing* because it was envisioned as prescribing nurses' actions.[8] In the 1970s, under the perceived pressures to define the domain of a nascent nursing discipline in the academy and to stake out the unique character of nursing research in competitions for funding (Risjord, 2011), the consensus view, of which Fawcett is an influential proponent, undermined the idea of practice-based theory.

Fawcett (2005) created a comprehensive and unified vision of basic nursing science that presupposes a production of abstract models and grand theories and their subsequent empirical testing (via the process of *theoretical substruction*). Fawcett clarifies that her "conceptual-theoretical-empirical formalization" permits "theory-generating research (bottom-up) or theory-testing (top-down) research" (Butts, 2012, p. 152). In her vision, all research in the discipline is connected, via the bottom-up or top-down processes, to a limited number of abstract theories unique to nursing. That is, only research that develops or tests *nursing* theory could be considered scientifically proper in nursing (Butts, 2012; Risjord, 2010, p. 26).

Against Borrowed Theory

We can appreciate how this stipulation of a unified nursing science as requiring all theoretical work in the discipline to flow from and/or to feed into its unique grand theories immediately discriminates against what has been dubbed "borrowed theory."[9] This position is untenable within the contemporary philosophy of science that posits the "explanatory coherence" view of theory. Theories are

> coherent sets of propositions, where coherence is generated by the relationship of questions to answers. Theoretical propositions are answers to questions about human problems or striking phenomena. These answers raise further questions, and the aim of scientific theorizing is to answer these questions in a systematic way.
>
> (Risjord, 2010, p. 119)

Thus, according to the coherence view, theories comprise not a pyramid but a web or a patchwork quilt (Risjord, 2010, p. 38). Postpositivist philosophers of science like Willard Van Orman Quine and Hilary Putnam rejected positivist beliefs about theories consisting of levels, distinct theories operating with unique concepts, theories independently supported by observation, and a theory–observation distinction (Risjord, 2010, p. 106).

Equipped with postpositivist insights, Risjord (2010) squarely criticizes nurses' rejection of borrowed theory. The prevailing nursing perspective saw the strength of nursing science in its unique theories and concepts. But this perspective is erroneous; it weakens nursing scholarship. For, "when a scientist draws on a theory that has been confirmed in another domain, she adds the empirical support of that domain to her view" (Risjord, 2010, p. 109). And further,

> to insist . . . that it [a theory from another discipline] be reformulated in novel nursing terms would be to cut off the support available from existing tests in a variety of domains. The theory would be made unique to nursing at the cost of its empirical validity.
>
> (Risjord, 2010, p. 109)

Science is concerned with the empirical validity of theories. If theory is imagined as a web or a quilt, it gets stronger when each thread or piece is connected to theories in other domains (Risjord, 2010).

What are the implications of this understanding of interdisciplinary theory for my argument? A prejudice against borrowed theory has likely been one of the most obvious obstacles to accepting theoretical ideas from outside nursing, most notably from the social sciences and the humanities (see also C. Holmes, 1991). At the extreme, to gain admission into "nursing science," theories from other disciplines needed to be thoroughly shaped into nursing's mould, as I illustrate in further chapters. This practice of "theoretical reformulation" can be profoundly problematic. The knotty character of "reformulation," of assimilating concepts from one theory into another, is underscored by the contemporary philosophy of science literature on the nature of concepts. Risjord (2010) asks, Are concepts "theory-formed" (i.e. their meaning is non-referential and depends on the context of use) or "theory-forming" (i.e. concepts treated as labels for objects or ideas, and developed at the outset, prior to connecting them into theoretical propositions)? In contrast to the latter understanding evident in influential American nursing theory literature that concepts are "building blocks" clarified prior to theory construction (e.g. Chinn & Jacobs, 1983; Chinn & Kramer, 2011, 2015; L. O. Walker & Avant, 2011), an answer agreed upon in contemporary philosophy is that concepts take their meaning from the theoretical context in which they operate (e.g. Manchester, 1986, p. 248; Paley, 2006, p. 278). Concepts are "theory-formed." Thus, a process of "theoretical reformulation," when concepts from "borrowed theory" are annexed to concepts of extant nursing theory, risks drastically changing the meaning of the (non-nursing) ideas.

Concluding Thoughts

In this chapter, I exposed key philosophical ideas founding American nursing theory and "unique" nursing science. I followed Mark Risjord's (2010) perceptive analysis of the metatheoretical debates that characterized a nascent nursing science. Risjord's critique reveals the deep and pervasive influence of mid-20th-century logical positivist philosophy of science on nursing science. Thus, nursing science is founded upon the following beliefs (Petrovskaya et al., 2019): scientific disciplines develop a unique, discipline-specific set of theories; a goal of scientific research lies in theory development and testing; theories necessarily include abstract and general laws; testing of theory presupposes deduction of hypotheses from the laws (a deductive-nomological, pyramid-like logical structure of theory); and science is value-free. This image guides some nurse scholars to treat any "borrowed theory," including continental philosophy, with caution and to reshape it in terms of extant nursing models. Into the first decade of 2000s, nursing academic discourse displayed combinations of these beliefs. American nursing theory literature (Table A2 in the Appendix) shows that nursing writings and genres loyal to one or another version of this framework (and that operate with particular formal terminology, i.e. conceptual framework, grand theory, middle-range theory,[10] practice-level theory, borrowed theory, metaparadigm, paradigms, concept development, or model[11] of knowledge development) were granted the status of "nursing knowledge" (see Haynes et al., 2004, p. 74, for a typical depiction of the structure of nursing knowledge in an introductory nursing text).

Moreover, this historically produced intellectual matrix seems to set the expectation that theoretical nursing writings should be rhetorically couched in the formalized language of the "unique nursing disciplinary structure" (for an example in relation to narrative theory, or "Story Theory," see Prufeta, 2014). I argue that these disciplinary theoretical practices established within the matrix of American nursing theory have hindered a fuller appreciation of French philosophy and other continentally influenced nursing theorizing. Continental and other social theory-informed scholarship, both non-American and some American (examples of which are presented in further chapters), *neither* operated with formal terminology such as grand theory, paradigms, or model of knowledge development, *nor* assumed such a matrix in the background. When a formal, "scientistic" conception of (American nursing) theory dominates nursing imagination and literature, both continental philosophy and some of the best examples of nursing theorizing become unintelligible (Petrovskaya et al., 2019).

Notes

1 Risjord's (2010) book was enthusiastically received by British philosophers working and writing in nursing (Edwards, 2011; Paley, 2010). They commented on Risjord's rigorous, respectful, and well-articulated critique and endorsed his argument. A Canadian professor of nursing, June Kikuchi (2014), although disagreeing that the question *What is nursing?* is empirical, unreservedly approved of Risjord's rejection of the notion of nursing as a basic science and commended his determination to ground nursing science in the values and problems of nursing practice.

In contrast, Clarke (2011) and Theodoridis (2018) levelled criticism against Risjord (2010). Clarke detected circularity in Risjord's argument: confusion about whether nursing will be strengthened by drawing on knowledge from other disciplines or by developing unique, intrinsic knowledge. In my reading of Risjord, he is clear in his position, supported by contemporary philosophy of science, that a web-like, explanatory coherence view of knowledge, which transgresses the boundaries of "unique" disciplines, trumps the logical positivist conception. It is tempting to suggest that Clarke in fact is sympathetic to the idea of the unique disciplinary knowledge. However, Clarke devoted only one page to a discussion of Risjord's argument and never openly confronted him on this issue. On the other hand, Clarke's overall argument had some commonalities with that of Risjord: "Nursing is a practice-based activity. . . . Transpersonal nursing models [i.e., the American grand theory] are particularly criticizable in respect of their unworldly character as are also concepts based on shallow usages of physics. . . . I argue that sensible measurements of the 'real world' are possible – without endorsing positivism – and that nursing requires little recourse to logically unsustainable claims" (Clarke, 2011, p. 403). Importantly, Clarke erroneously associated the developments in the field of nursing knowledge (i.e. "unworldly theory") with the influence of Foucault. He also blamed "continental philosophy" – not nurses' misrepresentation of it – for some nurse theorists' and researchers' excessive focus on "subjective meanings." Theodoridis (2018) disagreed with Risjord's (2010) analogy of standpoint feminism as a useful epistemological position for nurses. For the purpose of my argument, however, what matters is that no critic disputed Risjord's analysis of logical positivist influences on American nursing theory.

The aforementioned responses to Risjord's (2010) book originated from outside the United States, that is, from outside Risjord's field of analysis. Inside the United States, leading theoretical journals *Nursing Science Quarterly* and *Advances in Nursing Science*, as well as widely known textbooks on nursing theory – whose central assumptions about theory Risjord targeted – were silent about Risjord's work (e.g. Butts & Rich, 2014; Chinn & Kramer, 2011, 2015; Fitzpatrick & Whall, 2016; Meleis, 2012), have given it a tokenistic nod (e.g. Fitzpatrick & McCarthy, 2014, p. 6), or have shrugged off its concerns (e.g. L.O. Walker & Avant, 2011, p. 173, dismiss one of Risjord's earlier criticisms of an approach to concept analysis espoused by these authors). One exception might be *Philosophy of Science for Nursing Practice: Concepts and Application* (Dahnke & Dreher, 2011), which mentions Risjord's distinction between the theory–practice gap as a matter of translation versus relevance (p. 68). This lack of acknowledgement of important criticisms in our discipline has been previously noticed in relation to nursing phenomenology (Petrovskaya, 2014a, 2014b) and identified as an intellectual problem in nursing (David Allen, 2013).

2 The phrase *nursing science* has accrued a range of meanings in American nursing disciplinary literature. As I explain later in this chapter, most significant for my work is the distinction rarely made between what American nurse *theorists* call nursing science (and what Risjord examined in his book) and what nurse *scientists* (e.g. Gortner discussed in Chapter 4) and nurse researchers consider nursing science.

3 In this book, I do not make a rigorous philosophical distinction between the logical positivism outlined by Risjord (2010) and the logical empiricism outlined by Bluhm (2014). Importantly, too, I do not compare logical positivism and post-structuralism. In fact, I do not advance claims about logical positivism per se. Rather, I draw on Risjord's analysis of logical positivist influences in nursing to describe the matrix structuring reception of postmodernism, post-structuralism, and Foucault in American nursing theory.

4 I do not advocate a widely established convention, most notably in American and Canadian literature, to supplement the label "nursing science" with "nursing art." Rather, my position aligns with those objections to the conceptualizations of nursing professional practice as a science that do not seek to balance it with appeals to "art" (Edwards, 1999, 2001; Sellman, 2011; see also Drummond, 2004, p. 529; and selected articles by Rafferty).

5 Risjord (2010) elucidates only *philosophical* influences on nursing science; that is, he does not trace the sociological roots of nurses' conceptions of theory. Worth observing is the difference between a kind of sociology that informed American nursing science (i.e. sociological formal theory) and ethnomethodological sociology drawn upon by British-educated nurses (e.g. Davina Allen, Latimer, Purkis), whose writings easily integrated contemporary social theory such as post-structuralism.

6 Again, this was a logical positivist vision of science. Actual practices of those sciences did not necessarily coincide with this vision, as a historicist philosophy of science (and later, the sociological studies of science) demonstrated.

7 The contemporary philosophy of science alternatives to the pyramid model of theory are the "explanatory coherence" view of theory and inter-level scientific modelling. These approaches to theory evoke a metaphor of a web or a patchwork quilt (Risjord, 2010, p. 38)

8 The practice theorists disagreed on some issues: Wald and Leonard (1964) and Dickoff and James (1968) advocated unique theory. In contrast, Gunter (1962) and Ellis (1968) argued for an acceptance of theories from other disciplines, which would be developed and modified. Dickoff and James were influenced by Dewey's ideas; thus, they objected to the value neutrality of theory. However, their writings too exhibited some logical positivist traits like a theory–observation dichotomy (Risjord, 2011, pp. 496–497). Another caveat is that the label "practice theory" as used in American nursing theory is not identical with the use of this phrase in social sciences and some nursing theoretical scholarship. The latter often refers to ethnomethodology, actor network theory, and related sociologically informed field studies of nursing practice (e.g. Rudge, Purkis, Bjornsdottir, Davina Allen, Latimer).

9 A paradox: While claiming that borrowed theory is inconsistent with the nursing discipline, many American nurse theorists built their theories upon borrowed ideas like general systems theory, complexity theory, or phenomenology of Merlau-Ponty (Kim & Kollak, 2006; Sarter, 1988). In a sense, borrowed ideas were germane to nursing science.

10 Risjord (2010) points out important terminological conflation in nursing literature. Following the received view of theory, many nurse authors define middle-range theory as a middle layer in the hierarchy of scientific theory, between grand- and practice-based theories. Thus, middle-range theory is distinguished by its scope and abstraction. This view has been challenged in nursing literature by Lenz et al. (1995). They stated that the mid-range status depends not on scope or level of abstraction, but "on the adequacy of [theory's] empirical foundations" (p. 3). This distinction, crucial within the postpositivist philosophy of science, has been lost in nursing literature due to what Risjord dubs as Lenz et al.'s tactical error in the choice of terminology (Risjord, 2010, 2011, pp. 510–511).

11 Three conceptions of a model are discernible and often conflated in nursing literature. One, the logical positivist-influenced, is close to Fawcett's (2005) *conceptual model* and refers to one of the most abstract and general constructs – an "uninterpreted" theory. Another understanding of models refers to ways in which many nurse authors (e.g. Carter & Kulbok, 1995; Chinn & Kramer, 2015) seem to use the term: as a mind-map, heuristic device, or graphic presentation of main components of theory. Finally, some contemporary philosophers of science consider models *as* theories. Model-building is a primary approach in some natural sciences (Bluhm, 2014; Risjord, 2010). In these scientific models, specificity of factors is the key (see Crigger, 1996, for a nursing example). In itself, the second conception of *models* does not carry the assumptions of logical positivism. Research articles in *Advances in Nursing Science* often include models as a visual display of main components and as an organizing framework. However, the subtle presence of the received view of theory arises when discussions of these models are supported with references to the first view, as in Carter and Kulbok (1995).

References

Abbott, A. (1988). *The system of professions: An essay on the division of expert labor.* University of Chicago Press.

Allen, D. G. (1985). Nursing research and social control: Alternate models of science that emphasize understanding and emancipation. *Image: The Journal of Nursing Scholarship,* 17(2), 58–64.

Allen, D. G. (2013). David Allen. In A. Forss, C. Ceci, & J. S. Drummond (Eds.), *Philosophy of nursing: 5 questions* (pp. 1–5). Automatic Press/VIP.

Bluhm, R. L. (2014). The (dis)unity of nursing science. *Nursing Philosophy, 15*(4), 250–260.

Butts, J. B. (2012). The future of nursing: How important is discipline-specific knowledge? A conversation with Jacqueline Fawcett. Interview by Dr. Janie Butts and Dr. Karen Rich. *Nursing Science Quarterly, 25*(2), 151–154.

Butts, J. B., & Rich, K. L. (2014). *Philosophies and theories for advanced nursing practice* (2nd ed.). Jones & Bartlett Learning.

Carper, B. (1978). Fundamental patterns of knowing in nursing. *Advances in Nursing Science, 1*(1), 13–23.

Carter, K. F., & Kulbok, P. A. (1995). Evaluation of the interaction model of client health behavior through the first decade of research. *Advances in Nursing Science, 18*(1), 62–73.

Chinn, P. L. (1985). Debunking myths in nursing theory and research. *Image: The Journal of Nursing Scholarship, 17*(2), 45–49.

Chinn, P. L., & Jacobs, M. K. (1983). *Theory and nursing: A systematic approach.* Mosby.

Chinn, P. L., & Kramer, M. K. (2011). *Integrated theory and knowledge development in nursing* (8th ed.). Elsevier Mosby.

Chinn, P. L., & Kramer, M. K. (2015). *Knowledge development in nursing: Theory and process* (9th ed.). Elsevier Health Sciences.

Clarke, L. (2011). So what exactly is nursing knowledge? *Journal of Psychiatric & Mental Health Nursing, 18*(5), 403–410.

Conant, L. H. (1967). Closing the practice–theory gap. *Nursing Outlook, 15*(11), 37–39.

Crigger, N. I. (1996). Testing an uncertainty model for women with multiple sclerosis. *Advances in Nursing Science, 18*(3), 37–47.

Dahnke, M. D., & Dreher, H. M. (2011). *Philosophy of science for nursing practice: Concepts and application.* Springer Publishing Company.

Dickoff, J., & James, P. (1968). A theory of theories: A position paper. *Nursing Research, 17*(3), 197–203.

Diers, D. (1994). What is nursing? In J. McCloskey & H. K. Grace (Eds.), *Current issues in nursing* (4th ed., pp. 5–14). Mosby.

Dingwall, R. (1975). Accomplishing profession. *The Sociological Review, 24*(2), 331–349.

Donaldson, S. K. (2010). Preface. In M. Risjord (Ed.), *Nursing knowledge: Science, practice, and philosophy* (pp. xiii–xviii). Wiley-Blackwell.

Donaldson, S. K., & Crowley, D. M. (1978). The discipline of nursing. *Nursing Outlook, 26*(2), 113–120.

Drevdahl, D. (1999). Meanings of community in a community health center. *Public Health Nursing, 16*(6), 417–425.

Drummond, J. S. (2004). Nursing and the avant-garde. *International Journal of Nursing Studies, 41*(5), 525–533.

Dzurec, L. (1989). The necessity for and evolution of multiple paradigms for nursing research: A poststructuralist perspective. *Advances in Nursing Science, 11*(4), 69–77.

Edwards, S. D. (1999). The idea of nursing science. *Journal of Advanced Nursing, 29*(3), 563–569.

Edwards, S. D. (2001). *Philosophy of nursing: An introduction.* Palgrave.

Edwards, S. (2011). Book review. *Theoretical Medicine and Bioethics, 32*(2), 129–131.

Ellis, R. (1968). Characteristics of significant theories. *Nursing Research, 17*(3), 217–222.

Ellis, R. (1969). The practitioner as theorist. *American Journal of Nursing, 69*(7), 428–435.

Fawcett, J. (1997). The relationship between theory and research: A double helix. In L. H. Nicoll (Ed.), *Perspectives on nursing theory* (3rd ed., pp. 716–725). Lippincott. (Original work published in *Advances in Nursing Science, 1*(1), 49–62, in 1978)

Fawcett, J. (2005). *Contemporary nursing knowledge: Analysis and evaluation of nursing models and theories* (2nd ed.). F. A. Davis.

Fitzpatrick, J. J., & McCarthy, G. (Eds.). (2014). *Theories guiding nursing research and practice: Making nursing knowledge development explicit.* Springer Publishing Company.

Fitzpatrick, J. J., & Whall, A. L. (Eds.). (2016). *Conceptual models of nursing: Global perspectives* (5th ed.). Pearson.

Gibbs, J. P. (1994). Resistance in sociology to formal theory construction. In J. Hage (Ed.), *Formal theory in sociology: Opportunity or pitfall?* (pp. 90–103). SUNY Press.

Gortner, S. R. (1991). Historical development of doctoral programs: Shaping our expectations. *Journal of Professional Nursing, 7*(1), 45–53.

Gortner, S. R. (1997). Nursing's syntax revisited: A critique of philosophies said to influence nursing theories. In L. H. Nicoll (Ed.), *Perspectives on nursing theory* (3rd ed., pp. 357–368). Lippincott. (Original work published in *International Journal of Nursing Studies, 30*(6), 477–488, in 1993)

Gortner, S. R. (2000). Knowledge development in nursing: Our historical roots and future opportunities. *Nursing Outlook, 48*(2), 60–67.

Grace, H. (1978). The development of doctoral education in nursing: A historical perspective. In N. L. Chaska (Ed.), *The nursing profession: Views through the mist* (pp. 112–122). McGraw-Hill.

Gunter, L. M. (1962). Notes on a theoretical framework for nursing research. *Nursing Research, 11*(4), 219–222.

Hacking, I. (1983). *Representing and intervening: Introductory topics in the philosophy of natural science.* Cambridge University Press.

Hardy, M. E. (1978). Perspectives on nursing theory. *Advances in Nursing Science, 1*(1), 27–48.

Haynes, L., Butcher, H., & Boese, T. (2004). *Nursing in contemporary society: Issues, trends, and transition into practice.* Pearson Prentice Hall.

Holmes, C. A. (1991). Theory: Where are we going and what have we missed along the way? In G. Gray & R. Pratt (Eds.), *Towards a discipline of nursing* (pp. 435–460). Churchill Livingstone.

Hughes, E. C. (1963). Professions. *Daedalus, 92*(4), 655–668.

Hussey, T. (2001). Book review: Perspectives on philosophy of science in nursing. *Nursing Philosophy, 2,* 274–276.

Johnson, B. M., & Webber, P. B. (2010). *An introduction to theory and reasoning in nursing* (3rd ed.). Lippincott Williams & Wilkins.

Johnson, D. E. (1959). The nature of a science of nursing. *Nursing Outlook, 7*(5), 291–294.

Kikuchi, J. F. (2014). Risjord's philosophy of nursing science: Concerns and questions. *Nursing Philosophy, 15*(1), 46–49.

Kim, H. S., & Kollak, I. (Eds.). (2006). *Nursing theories: Conceptual and philosophical foundations* (2nd ed.). Springer Publishing Company.

Larsen, J., & Baumgart, A. J. (1992). Introduction to nursing in Canada. In A. J. Baumgart & J. Larsen (Eds.), *Canadian nursing faces the future* (2nd ed., pp. 3–21). Mosby Year Book.

Laudan, L. (1999). Dissecting the holist picture of scientific change. In E. C. Polifroni & M. Welch (Eds.), *Perspectives on philosophy of science in nursing: An historical and contemporary anthology* (pp. 105–125). Lippincott Williams & Wilkins. (Original work published 1984)

Lenz, E. R., Suppe, F., Gift, A. G., Pugh, L. C., & Milligan, R. A. (1995). Collaborative development of middle-range nursing theories: Toward a theory of unpleasant symptoms. *Advances in Nursing Science, 17*(3), 1–13.

Liaschenko, J. (1994). The moral geography of home care. *Advances in Nursing Science, 17*(2), 16–26.

Liaschenko, J. (1997). Ethics and the geography of the nurse–patient relationship: Spatial vulnerabilities and gendered space. *Scholarly Inquiry for Nursing Practice, 11*(1), 45–59.

Liaschenko, J., & Fisher, A. (1999). Theorizing the knowledge that nurses use in the conduct of their work. *Scholarly Inquiry for Nursing Practice, 13*(1), 29–41.

Liaschenko, J., & Peter, E. (2004). Nursing ethics and conceptualizations of nursing: Profession, practice and work. *Journal of Advanced Nursing, 46*(5), 488–495.

Manchester, P. (1986). Analytic philosophy and foundational inquiry: The method. In P. L. Munhall & C. J. Oiler (Eds.), *Nursing research: A qualitative perspective* (pp. 229–249). Appleton-Century-Crofts.

Markie, P. (2015). Rationalism vs. empiricism. In E. N. Zalta (Ed.), *The Stanford encyclopedia of philosophy.* http://plato.stanford.edu/entries/rationalism-empiricism/

McCloskey, J., & Grace, H. K. (Eds.). (1994). *Current issues in nursing* (4th ed.). Mosby.

Meleis, A. I. (1997). *Theoretical nursing: Development and progress* (3rd ed.). Lippincott.

Meleis, A. I. (2012). *Theoretical nursing: Development and progress* (5th ed.). Wolters Kluwer/Lippincott Williams & Wilkins.

Munhall, P. L. (1982). Nursing philosophy and nursing research: In apposition or opposition? *Nursing Research, 31*(3), 176–177, 181.

Newman, M. A. (1972). Nursing's theoretical evolution. *Nursing Outlook, 20*(7), 449–453.

Paley, J. (2006). Book review: Nursing theorists and their work. *Nursing Philosophy, 7*(4), 275–280.

Paley, J. (2010). Book review. Nursing knowledge: Science, practice, and philosophy. *Nursing Philosophy, 11*(3), 216–219.

Petrovskaya, O. (2014a). Is there nursing phenomenology after Paley? Essay on rigorous reading. *Nursing Philosophy, 15*(1), 60–71.

Petrovskaya, O. (2014b). Domesticating Paley: How we misread Paley (and phenomenology). *Nursing Philosophy, 15*(1), 72–75.

Petrovskaya, O., Purkis, M. E., & Bjornsdottir, K. (2019). Revisiting "intelligent nursing": Olga Petrovskaya in conversation with Mary Ellen Purkis and Kristin Bjornsdottir. *Nursing Philosophy, 20*(3). https://doi-org.ezproxy.library.uvic.ca/10.1111/nup.12259

Prufeta, P. (2014). Story theory. In J. J. Fitzpatrick & G. McCarthy (Eds.), *Theories guiding nursing research and practice: Making nursing knowledge development explicit* (pp. 239–250). Springer Publishing Company.

Reed, P. (1995). A treatise on nursing knowledge development for the 21st century: Beyond postmodernism. *Advances in Nursing Science, 17*(3), 70–84.

Risjord, M. (2010). *Nursing knowledge: Science, practice, and philosophy.* Wiley-Blackwell.

Risjord, M. (2011). Nursing science. In F. Gifford (Ed.), *Philosophy of medicine* (pp. 489–522). Elsevier.

Rodgers, B. L. (2005). *Developing nursing knowledge: Philosophical traditions and influences.* Lippincott Williams & Wilkins.

Ross Kerr, J. (1996). Professionalization in Canadian nursing. In J. Ross Kerr & J. MacPhail (Eds.), *Canadian nursing: Issues and perspectives* (3rd ed., pp. 23–30). Mosby.

Sandelowski, M. (1999). Troubling distinctions: A semiotics of the nursing/technology relationship. *Nursing Inquiry, 6*(3), 198–207.

Sandelowski, M. (2000). *Devices and desires: Gender, technology, and American nursing.* University of North Carolina Press.

Sarter, B. (1988). Philosophical sources of nursing theory. *Nursing Science Quarterly, 1*(2), 52–59.

Schlotfeldt, R. M. (1960). Reflections on nursing research. *American Journal of Nursing, 60*(4), 492–494.

Sellman, D. (2011). *What makes a good nurse.* Jessica Kingsley Publishers.

Silva, M. C., & Rothbart, D. (1997). An analysis of changing trends in philosophies of science on nursing theory development and testing. In L. H. Nicoll (Ed.), *Perspectives on nursing theory* (3rd ed., pp. 293–306). Lippincott. (Original work published in *Advances in Nursing Science, 6*(2), 1–13, in 1984)

Slevin, O. (2003). An epistemology of nursing: Ways of knowing and being. In L. Basford & O. Slevin (Eds.), *Theory and practice of nursing: An integrated approach to caring practice* (2nd ed., pp. 143–171). Nelson Thornes.

Theodoridis, K. (2018). Nursing as concrete philosophy, Part I: Risjord on nursing knowledge. *Nursing Philosophy, 19*(2), 1–8, e12205.

Uebel, T. (2014). Vienna circle. In E. N. Zalta (Ed.), *The Stanford encyclopedia of philosophy.* http://plato.stanford.edu/archives/spr2014/entries/vienna-circle/

van Fraassen, B. (1999a). Arguments concerning scientific realism. In E. C. Polifroni & M. Welch (Eds.), *Perspectives on philosophy of science in nursing: An historical and contemporary anthology* (pp. 88–104). Lippincott Williams & Wilkins. (Original work published 1980)

van Fraassen, B. (1999b). The pragmatics of explanation. In E. C. Polifroni & M. Welch (Eds.), *Perspectives on philosophy of science in nursing: An historical and contemporary anthology* (pp. 166–178). Lippincott Williams & Wilkins. (Original work published 1980)

Wald, F. S., & Leonard, R. C. (1964). Towards development of nursing practice theory. *Nursing Research, 13*(4), 309–313.

Walker, L. O. (1971). Toward a clearer understanding of the concept of nursing theory. *Nursing Research, 20*(5), 428–435.

Walker, L. O., & Avant, K. C. (2011). *Strategies for theory construction in nursing* (5th ed.). Pearson Prentice Hall.

Watson, J. (1995). Postmodernism and knowledge development in nursing. *Nursing Science Quarterly, 8*(2), 60–64.

Webster, G., Jacox, A., & Baldwin, B. (1981). Nursing theory and the ghost of the received view. In H. K. Grace & J. C. McCloskey (Eds.), *Current issues in nursing.* Blackwell Scientific Publications.

Winther, R. G. (2015). The structure of scientific theories. In E. N. Zalta (Ed.), *The Stanford encyclopedia of philosophy.* http://plato.stanford.edu/entries/structure-scientific-theories/

Yeo, M. (1989). Integration of nursing theory and nursing ethics. *Advances in Nursing Science, 11*(3), 33–42.

4 Postmodern and Post-structural Ideas in American Nursing Texts I

Gortner, Dzurec, Reed, Watson, and *Nursing Science Quarterly*

Many readers, especially outside the United States, may think that American nursing theory is a thing of the past, once prominent in disciplinary discourse but put aside as unconvincing or replaced by new subject areas in busy nursing curricula. While this is often the case, nursing theory maintains its noticeable presence, for example, through nursing theory conferences in the United States. Perspectives on unique nursing science and discipline-specific theories articulated by various scholars are not identical. They present nursing science from varying angles – sometimes opposing – but invariably within the intellectual matrix whose recognizable features were addressed in the previous chapter. Their commonalities stem from the convoluted logical-positivist influences, as Risjord (2010) demonstrated.

In the 1990s and later, these perspectives were maintained by regular editions of long-running textbooks including portraits of nurse theorists and descriptions and examples of their work (Alligood, 2014, 2018; Alligood & Tomey, 2010; Tomey & Alligood, 1998, 2002, 2006); conceptual models and middle-range theories (Fitzpatrick & McCarthy, 2014; Fitzpatrick & Whall, 2005, 2016; M. Parker, 2006; M. Parker & M. C. Smith, 2010; M. J. Smith & Liehr, 2014); the integrated view of nursing knowledge based on "patterns of knowing" (Chinn & Kramer, 2004, 2008, 2011, 2015, 2019); guides to theory construction (B. Johnson & Webber, 2010; L. O. Walker & Avant, 2005, 2011); anthologies of (meta) theoretical publications (Cody, 2006; Kenney, 1996, 2002; Nicoll,1997; Reed & Shearer, 2009, 2012; Roy & Jones, 2007); and compendiums of "contemporary nursing knowledge" (Fawcett, 2005; Meleis, 1997, 2007, 2012). This textual production sustains an established field of "theoretical nursing knowledge" and perpetuates particular views of nursing science, nursing knowledge, and theory, as delineated in the preceding chapter.

In this and the following chapter, I undertake a detailed examination of the American nursing literature citing postmodern and post-structural ideas roughly during the first two decades of nursing's encounter with these French philosophical currents. As noted previously, the influence of postmodernism and post-structuralism on American nursing scholarship is noticeably less prominent than on Australian, British, and Canadian nursing scholarship. Despite heterogeneity in how postmodern and post-structural ideas were applied in American nursing publications (Tables A1 and A2), it is possible to discern recurring practices

DOI: 10.4324/9781003194439-4

of knowledge production that afford greater visibility to certain ways of reading postmodern and post-structural work, while rendering other ideas undesirable and unintelligible.

I argue that to the degree that postmodern and post-structural ideas are shaped to conform to the existing image of "unique nursing science," they are made visible, that is, embraced within nursing theoretical discourses. However, this visibility comes with a price: highly selective reading and a compromised integrity of continental ideas. On the other hand, theorizing informed by postmodern and post-structural theory that does *not* utilize the formal and rhetorical resources of "nursing science" (i.e. language of "levels of theory," "paradigms," "borrowed theory") and does not share the ideological aims of the latter (i.e. an endorsement of a "holistic nurse" as a preferable ethical persona; the professionalization project; advancement of nursing's metanarrative in place of metanarratives of "medical model" and "traditional science") remains unintelligible, as it were, and outside of the "nursing theory/nursing knowledge" domain, as my survey of authoritative textbooks listed earlier reveals.

In Chapters 4 and 5, I use examples of American nursing writings citing Foucault and/or claiming postmodern or post-structural perspectives. These examples are mostly drawn from a comprehensive (to the best of my knowledge) pool of American academic nursing literature from the first two decades of the nursing's encounter with these French theories (Tables A1 and A2). The question that guides my analysis is, In what ways have these authors reacted to or incorporated postmodern and post-structural ideas? I will elucidate the positions of individual nurse scholars and theoretical nursing journals. To understand these scholars' and journals' deployment of postmodern and post-structural thinking, I provide relevant intellectual context. In some cases, as with the work of Pamela Reed, unravelling her ideas requires several pages. In other cases, my writing is concise: Whenever well-informed and relevant criticisms of postmodern nursing writings already exist that corroborate my observations – as with Jean Watson's work – I draw on these criticisms. (As explained in the introduction, one of the goals of my study is to highlight important but ignored or dismissed criticisms that question established truths of nursing disciplinary discourses.) My discussion presents contrasting or overlapping discursive positions carved out within the matrix of American nursing science. Within those discursive positions, what sense could be, and has been, made of postmodern and post-structural ideas? In turn, what are those approaches to theorizing in our discipline and ways of reading Foucault that are less visible and teeter on the edge of intelligibility within the matrix of American nursing theory?

Susan Gortner's "Nursing's Syntax Revisited: A Critique of Philosophies Said to Influence Nursing Theories," 1993: Foucault as a Philosopher of the Month

Although Susan Gortner mentions Foucault only once – dismissingly – I chose to present her position at length. As an American scholar promoting rigorous biological and behavioural research in nursing, she was concerned with a proliferation of what some nurse authors proposed as alternative "scientific paradigms" (namely, phenomenology, critical theory, and feminism) in nursing theoretical literature. My aim in starting with Gortner's writings is to suggest that insistence on linking broad theoretical writings on the nature of nursing – especially those informed by social theoretical and continental philosophical ideas – with the project of nursing *science* (understood in a specific way in American nursing theory) has foreclosed or delayed possibilities for engaging with continental philosophy as the object of the humanities. Beginning with Gortner's writings also helps to unearth contradictory meanings of the notion *nursing science* in American academic nursing.

So closely have the notions of "nursing science" and "nursing theory" intertwined in the American discourse of "disciplinary nursing knowledge" circulated through multiple editions of theory textbooks and through the journals *Advances in Nursing Science* and *Nursing Science* Quarterly,[1] that it is perhaps difficult to recognize the existence of alternative conceptions and practices of nursing *science*. In fact, this latter conception of nursing science predates the consensus view of science and theory of the 1970s sustained by the nursing theory literature and can be traced back to the vision of science that underpinned the Nurse Scientist program of the 1960s, when U.S. federal funding enabled nurses to train as researchers in biological and behavioural sciences (Gortner, 1991, 2000). Susan Gortner, a professor of nursing at the University of California at San Francisco from 1978 to 1994 (died in 2006), was the first nurse scientist to serve in the late 1960s and early 1970s in the federal agency that supported nursing research (Gortner, 1991, 2000). Her scientific background as a nurse-researcher in the field of cardiology and her understanding of interdisciplinary scientific research have informed her perspective and writings on nursing science. Gortner's perspective, aligned with the postpositivist philosophy of science as a critique of logical positivism – a view that reflected many other nurse researchers' (as opposed to some nurse theoreticians') understanding of science throughout the 1980s and 1990s – has been out of sync with the consensus view.

The consensus view, as Risjord (2010) demonstrated, is thoroughly grounded in the logical positivist philosophy of science but does not recognize this influence. This creates a challenge for the reader wishing to excavate *alternative* views of nursing science. Indeed, how can the alternative be identified if both the consensus view and its alternative energetically reject logical positivism? The well-known metatheoretical and theoretical nursing literature that *denies* logical positivism and rhetorically distances itself from this outdated philosophy, in fact, according to Risjord, *exemplifies* positivist influences. The features of "positivistic" philosophy that are commonly castigated in nursing literature are reductionism, realism, objectivity, and quantification. These features are said to characterize biomedical and behavioural research. Although Gortner is explicitly *postpositivist* in her discussions of science and her choice of sources, and she points out that it is erroneous to associate "quantification" with positivism (Schumacher & Gortner, 1992), her empirical focus, her assumption of reality as an essential ground for scientific activity, and her advocacy for the biological-behavioural research have positioned her squarely in the "positivist camp," an adversary of unique nursing science.

An essential ingredient of the lack of congruence between Gortner's position and the consensus view of nursing science was Gortner's high esteem for practice theory. She writes, "The field of practice must figure prominently as the empirical source of many theoretical models, and as the setting for their subsequent verification" (Gortner, 1975/1997, p. 695). However, what she observes in nursing is far from her expectation: "The empirical work and the theoretical or rational work (the development of theory) occurred on parallel and nonintersecting planes" (Gortner, 1983/1997, p. 292). Research in nursing as a practice profession should be guided by a question: What are the outcomes of nursing care for patients? "Note the key words," Gortner (1975/1997) writes, describing her vision of nursing science, "patient and effect. This is the critical nucleus of patient care research" (p. 696). Gortner's advocacy for empirical, practice-informed theory positioned her unfavourably on a theoretical stage dominated by grand theory.

No surprise, Gortner was reluctant to grant the status of science to the abstract theoretical activity that arose in nursing from the 1970s. In 1999, Gortner gave a keynote address at the 50th Anniversary of the School of Nursing at the University of California at Los Angeles about the past and future of knowledge development in nursing (Gortner, 2000). It is striking how the history of nursing science she presented, if contrasted with the history familiar to nurses through the "American nursing theory" literature, sounds as if they were histories of two different, minimally overlapping disciplines! Her seven-page overview of the milestones of nursing science includes *two sentences* on what many consider the preferred, or even the only, story of nursing science:

> With this momentum and influx of prepared scientist nurses, some of whom had been exposed to philosophers in their graduate programs, came debate about the nature of nursing science, what should be the prevailing world view and research approach. We spent a great deal of time speaking and writing to empiricism, phenomenology (later hermeneutics), critical theory, and feminism, to name but a few. Postpositivists, of which I am one, were maligned for speaking to the components of "good science" such as credibility, reproducibility, and rigor.
>
> (Gortner, 2000, p. 64)

Conspicuously, no mention of "nursing theory" or "conceptual models" is made. Naming journals launched in 1978, she mentions only two, *Research in Nursing and Health* and *The Western Journal of Nursing Research*, leaving out the leading theoretical journal, *Advances in Nursing Science*. Earlier, Gortner (1980/1997) distinguished science, "the body of codified understanding of the natural universe and of human social and individual behavior," from research, "the tool of science" (p. 266). Yet, as she makes clear in her keynote, to talk about nursing science means to talk about nursing research that contributed significantly to solve problems encountered in clinical nursing practice (Gortner, 2000). Gortner's depiction contrasts with the following logical positivist conception of science: "the body of scientific knowledge [as] the product includ[ing] scientific terminology and definitions, propositions, hypotheses, theories, and laws. . . [that] articulat[e] the logical foundations of scientific knowledge" (Silva & Rothbart, 1984/1997, pp. 296–297). Opposing this logical positivist understanding of science as a hierarchical, foundational structure of elements at differing levels of abstraction – an understanding that surreptitiously took root in nursing theoretical discourse – Gortner offered a counter-voice questioning nursing's "scientific" directions.

In the 1980s, American nursing theory rejected "traditional science" with its scientific method in favour of holistic, idealist, and subjective nursing theory and philosophy and phenomenological research (Gortner, 1990/1997; Paley, 2002). In short, "science [was] cast against humanism and hermeneutics" (Gortner, 1990/1997, p. 200). The humanistic focus of nursing was thought to be threatened by and incompatible with the scientific method (e.g. Munhall, 1982). Gortner (1983/1997) responded: "I argue against the position that research methods must be compatible with disciplinary philosophy, whatever that is. No other profession has had such a stringent requirement" (p. 292). Without controversy, the nursing profession espouses humanistic values of caring. But a belief that nursing's philosophy should guide and direct research strategy is misguided, Gortner (1990/1997, 1993/1997) rightly insisted.[2]

Gortner (1993/1997; Schumacher & Gortner, 1992) attempted to convince her opponents that contemporary empiricism was not what they thought it was, that it had moved past logical positivism and already operated on a plane of assumptions claimed desirable in nursing science. Postpositivist science is non-foundational as it rejects absolute sources of knowledge. It embraces values, positing that there are no theory-neutral facts. Both quantitative and qualitative data are valid forms of evidence. Scientific realism accepts *unobservable* entities posited in scientific theories as real (i.e. the "metaphysical turn" in the philosophy of science). An emphasis has shifted from verification, or a concern with the origin and foundation of knowledge, to justification of knowledge claims, that is, evaluation of evidence brought to bear on them. Many postpositivists recognize that the belief in universal laws is erroneous. With these arguments, Gortner attempted to rectify misconceptions about science.

According to Gortner (1990/1997, 1993/1997), these misconceptions in nursing metatheoretical literature lead to extreme subjectivism promoted through the so-called alternative scientific paradigms, which she sets out to interrogate. In addition to phenomenology and hermeneutics, the alternative paradigms include critical theory and feminist ideas, all introduced into American nursing literature from the 1980s onwards. Gortner's (1990/1997) engagement with these relatively novel ideas touches upon the possibilities they offer; for example, hermeneutics assist in the "intersubjective consensual validation [of meaning] by participants" (p. 202), whereas critical theory applies to "situations of social interaction involving authority and power" (p. 203). Foucault figures only tangentially in Gortner's (1993/1997) writings when she dubs him a "philosopher of the month"

(p. 362), alongside Kuhn, Laudan, Habermas, and Toulmin, and identifies these philosophers' ideas as partially responsible for nurses' misunderstanding of contemporary empiricism.

The bulk of her discussion, however, revolves around concerns legitimate within the framework of Western science (to which many nurse theorists appealed as well): Without scrutiny by the community of scientists, how can we accept "self-understandings and self-theories . . . as warranted evidence and thus as measures of 'truth'"? (Gortner, 1990/1997, p. 201). Can understanding facilitated by a hermeneutic analysis be taken as the sole criterion for explanation? (p. 203). Understanding is indispensable for the clinician, but the goal of science is to provide prescription for practice. Thus, explanation should be grounded in causal inference. Explanation remains one of the foundational premises of science. Some feminist writers advocate "knowing through intimate attending" (Gortner, 1990/1997, p. 203), but the scientific requirement of generalizability and reproducibility highlights the limitations of this idiosyncratic "knowing."

It is within this context of nursing metatheoretical discussions, when continental ideas including those introduced by Foucault were presented as alternative *scientific paradigms*, that Gortner's (1993/1997) unsympathetic reaction should be placed. For science is already self-correcting, and any purported advantages of the "new science" are unconvincing for Gortner. Above all, Gortner (1990/1997, 1993/1997) writes that as *substitutes for scientific method*, critical theory, feminism, and phenomenology/hermeneutics, praised as subjective and idiographic, are unsatisfactory in terms of meeting the assumptions of scientific realism (research findings refer to the real world and may or may not be true) and explanatory power (not only accounting for a given event but generalizing to other events of the same set).[3] I suggest that Gortner's well-informed criticism of "nursing science" and its alternative paradigms is not directed at continental philosophy. It is rather the case that nursing literature stretched continental philosophical ideas too far from their original context – for example, posited them as a substitute for the scientific method. Then what Gortner is opposing in her writings is not continental philosophy per se but a presentation of continental philosophy as a substitute for the scientific method.

Although Gortner mentioned Foucault only in passing, I presented her position at length. As a scholar promoting rigorous biological and behavioural research in nursing, she was concerned with a proliferation of alternative "scientific paradigms" in nursing theoretical literature. Foucault's work was to be avoided because it signalled the postmodern relativization of scientific truth. We will see below that other nurses, who also extracted this idea from Foucault's work, have done so from completely different theoretical positions and put postmodern ideas to different uses. Gortner's work is interesting for another reason as well: She participated eruditely in both – largely non-overlapping – conversations in academic nursing, that of "traditional science" (used as a belittling term in nursing theory literature) and "nursing science/nursing theory." At the very least, Gortner's treatment of Foucault and other continental philosophers raises a question about the benefits, for the discipline of nursing, of presenting continental philosophy as an alternative *scientific* modality as opposed to an evolving theoretical conversation in the humanities (including the latter's criticisms of science, be it medical science or nursing science).

Laura C. Dzurec's "The Necessity for and Evolution of Multiple Paradigms for Nursing Research: A Post-structuralist Perspective," 1989

Laura Dzurec sought to address American metatheoretical debates, which in the 1980s focused on the types of "knowing" and "paradigms of science" suitable for the discipline. Conflicting perspectives of "positivism" and "phenomenology" can be reconciled, Dzurec (1989) suggested, by casting them, respectively, as dominant and subjugated knowledges à la Foucault. In this way, novel phenomenological, qualitative nursing research can be recognized on a par with well-established quantitative research. Dzurec's call for a diversity of nursing scholarship struck a chord with some Canadian nurse academics who rejected the methodological and theoretical divisiveness in the American academy (Stajduhar et al., 2001; Thorne et al., 1998, 2004) and advocated "critical multiplism" instead (Letourneau & M. Allen, 1999).

Dzurec's (1989) publication was the first to draw on post-structuralism and Foucault's notion of knowledge/power in American nursing literature. This article has been favourably commented upon for both its endorsement of intellectual pluralism and its foregrounding of a post-structural perspective. Consequently, her contributions appeared in edited textbooks, for example, *In Search of Nursing Science* (Omery et al., 1995) and an anthology *Perspectives on Philosophy of Science in Nursing* (Polifroni & Welch, 1999). Turning our attention to the format of the textbook, which can be treated as a monument to ideas recognized and accepted as the most important and lasting in the discipline, I should note that these American texts were the earliest to include sections explicitly labelled "postmodern philosophy of science" in nursing.

One uniting feature of these textbooks is their firm positioning of postmodern and other continental philosophy in the realm of *science* (a rather problematic undertaking brought to the reader's attention in my analysis of Gortner's work). The other commonality between these texts is the display of a commendable spectrum of theoretical/philosophical perspectives in nursing science – empiricism, pragmatism, phenomenology and hermeneutics, feminisms, critical theory, and post-structuralism – without attempting to reduce or synthesize these perspectives under the rubric of "distinctive disciplinary knowledge." Admittedly, however, the goal pursued by Polifroni and her co-authors (Packard & Polifroni, 1991/1999) is to move the discipline closer to an identification of "a fundamental question" (p. 503) or "THE central question in the science of nursing" (p. 505, capitals in original) – a project echoing the ambitions of the consensus view of unique nursing science.

Polifroni and Welch's (1999) anthology includes three articles addressing postmodernism: Dzurec (1989), Reed (1995), and Watson (1995). The latter two papers became American classics of "postmodern nursing science," oft cited in journals and books and repeatedly anthologized. As such, they continue to set the stage of what counts as postmodern theory within the discourse of theoretical nursing knowledge. It is to these two nurse authors that I now turn.

Pamela Reed's "A Treatise on Nursing Knowledge Development for the 21st Century: Beyond Postmodernism," 1995

Pamela Reed, a professor of nursing at the University of Arizona, is known for her writings on knowledge development in nursing as well as her role as the lead editor for the anthology *Perspectives on Nursing Theory* (Reed & Shearer, 2009, 2012). She is the author of the middle-range theory of self-transcendence (e.g. in Fitzpatrick & McCarthy, 2014). How does Reed envision scientific theory? The image of nursing theory assumed in her writings resembles the pyramid-like structure of nursing knowledge described by Risjord (2010). The metaparadigm concepts determining nursing's unique domain, levels of theory based on their abstractness, and scientific explanation consisting in subsuming empirical observations under a higher-level theory are recurrent themes throughout her work (Reed, 1995, 2006a, 2006b, 2008). In another publication, Reed describes a process of a "deductive reformulation using developmental theories" (Reed, 1991), which approximates steps of logical deduction of theoretical propositions from higher-level theories. In short, the pyramid structure of theory – a legacy of logical positivist philosophy of science (Risjord, 2010) – permeates Reed's perspective on nursing knowledge.

In contrast to those scholars who envision the growth of nursing knowledge primarily through grand theories, however, Reed's focus has consistently been on "practice-based theory" (Reed, 1996, 2006a, 2008) and "practitioner as theorist" (Reed, 2008). What is meant by "practitioner as theorist"? Reed articulates a "model of knowledge production" originating not with an academic theoretician but with a nurse in clinical practice. Her assertion, "to theorize is to think abstractly and make links between the empirical and conceptual" (Reed, 2006a, p. 37), is quite uncontroversial on the face of it. To produce a theory, "the nurse applies creative insight and knowledge to generate and prioritize potential explanations for the problem at hand. . . . [T]he experience or observation occurs first, followed by generation of hypotheses or potential explanations" (Reed, 2008, p. 319). That is, having obtained data from patient interactions, a practitioner should "integrate theoretical thinking with [these] data . . . to develop knowledge" (Reed, 2006a, p. 37). And another iteration of Reed's ideas:

> The nurse's observations become the fundamental theoretical units, which are spiraled up drawing in relevant theories. Theoretical explanations are then *peeled out* from what the nurse has observed. The resulting theory is applied, tested, and transformed into nursing knowledge in the crucible of nursing practice.
>
> (Reed, 2008, p. 316; italics in original)

Embedded in this vision are assumptions about the empirical observation as separate from and prior to any conceptual/theoretical frame, about the source of "the conceptual," and about the form a final product should take.

Reed's first assumption, a fact-theory distinction, was challenged by the well-known humanbecoming[4] scholars Gail Mitchell and Debra Bournes (2006) on the pages of *Nursing Science Quarterly*. Mitchell and Bournes rejected a possibility of "atheoretical practice" implied by Reed's insistence that "observation occurs first" and then theoretical knowledge is "peeled out from practice." Practice always already reflects implicit or explicit "values, culture, and conceptual thinking" (p. 117), argued Mitchell and Bournes. In her rejoinders, Reed does not directly address this challenge, although elsewhere Reed (1995, 1996, 2000) too emphasizes the shift in the philosophy of science from value-neutral to value-laden observations (i.e. a refutation of the possibility of atheoretical "facts").

In relation to the form that a theory should take, Reed seems to suggest the following: "up the spiral" thinking is a requirement, which leads to a nursing theory "at some level of [abstraction]" (Reed, 2006a, p. 37). This indicates that Reed does not depart from the pyramid image of science, only that she advocates theories at the lower level of abstraction, peeled out from practice and then possibly worked up the ladder of abstraction. A further caveat is that the metaparadigm concepts (the crown of the pyramid) and paradigms, or philosophy of nursing, play an important role in Reed's vision of theory supposedly derived from practice. Reed (1995, 2006b) appears to suggest that "the concepts" from the "extant theoretical and conceptual models" such as Martha Rogers's science, function as "the corrective" for the kinds of "facts" that can be legitimately drawn from practice in a process of theorizing. In this way, their philosophical differences notwithstanding, both Reed's *practice-based theory* and Mitchell and Bournes's *practice-guiding grand theory* authorize what a practitioner and/or theorist can *think/see*: Sifted through the conceptual net of extant nursing theory, will not the "facts" of nursing practice be predetermined? (For example, accounts of nursing practice generated in light of M. Rogers's science of *unitary human being* will be conducted in terms of energy fields.) Most notably, will not these ostensibly practice-based accounts/theories be stripped of "the social" (e.g. a non-romantic view of the nurse–patient interaction and an organizational context) that intrudes into nursing practice but is excluded by the "extant" American theoretical frameworks the nurse scientists are advised to use (Drevdahl, 1999a; Purkis, 1994, 2003)?[5]

Reed's position on the role of postmodernism in nursing diverges from the more stringent one that treats interdisciplinary theory with great caution, as a potential threat for nursing's unique field. For Reed, continuous nursing knowledge development and what she refers to as *the clarification of philosophical foundations of nursing science* depend on the ability of nurse scholars to recognize paradigmatic shifts in broader philosophical thinking and to revisit or undertake a "reformulation" of extant nursing knowledge. Therefore, she spearheads the idea of a critical examination of the scientific ideals in light of postmodern challenges. In Reed's application, however, these challenges do not trouble the established conception of "nursing science," theory, and practice.

Reed uses the term "postmodernism" in several articles (1996, 2006b, 2008), starting from the 1995, "A Treatise on Nursing Knowledge Development for the 21st Century: Beyond Postmodernism." Citing social science literature on postmodernism, in addition to Foucault and Lyotard, Reed (1995) lists postmodern novelties: a rejection of a single meaning of reality; an incredulity towards grand theories and other metanarratives; a suspicion towards truth and progress; a coupling of knowledge ("meaning") and power; a denial of an essence of human beings; and the dissolution of universals (p. 71). The word "deconstruction" appears on the list along with platitudes that "the focus of study is text" and "meaning derives from the relationship between the text and the reader" (p. 72). This sketch of "postmodern theory," although not uncommon in nursing and other professional disciplines, is unhelpfully broad-ranging and too superficial to provide an adequate snapshot of specific concepts. Claiming to draw on the work of American pragmatist philosopher Richard Rorty, Reed concludes her survey of postmodernism by positing the "shift from concern over the truth of one's findings to concern over the practical significance of the findings" (p. 72).

Reed's (1995) new "framework for knowledge development" for the 21st century includes important components with potentially wide appeal in nursing. In the spirit of postmodernism, she calls to "transcend the . . . dichotomies" of "research and practice, inductive and deductive reasoning, qualitative and quantitative data" (p. 72). She observes that the schisms between scientific inquiry, nursing philosophy, and practice are problematic, and the framework aims to link them, just as she suggested practice-based theory as a mechanism for uniting nursing theory and practice. Reed appeals to "postmodern thought" in order to "blur . . . the distinction between the nonempirical and empirical, theory and fact" (p. 74). What do these aspirations amount to? Reed undertakes a series of "reformulations" aimed at "broadening" the notion of the empirical: The *new empirical* affirms "personal stories" on a par with "biologic indicators" and legitimizes nursing's "nonempirical conceptual innovations" such as Margaret Newman's and Dorothea Orem's theories as examples of empirical scientific work (p. 74). Further, she identifies that the postmodern influences on the philosophy of science call for a critical examination of the nurse scientist's assumptions. "But critique alone is not enough," Reed (1995, p. 75) adds immediately after suggesting the usefulness of critical reflection. Following this statement, the next section of the article has a subheading: "Beyond the Critique: A Neomodernist View." Rather than accepting the postmodern challenges and questioning modernist ideas "about high theory or universal ideals" (p. 76), Reed seeks to modify modernism within a new framework of neomodernism.

Reed (1995) alludes to the common contention that postmodernism is nonnormative and thus cannot serve as a substantive foundation for the nursing profession and a discipline. This limitation – that the postmodern "critique [of nursing science] cannot serve as its own external corrective" (Reed, 1995, p. 75) – is perceived as deeply problematic by Reed. She proposes a solution: "The nursing scientist's critique process [should] be linked to a substantive overarching 'ideal' or metanarrative" (p. 75). In this way, nursing's "perspectives and values . . . that distinguish nursing knowledge and the caring application of that knowledge" (p. 76) are preserved. She names two "metanarratives," nursing philosophy and nursing practice, as regulating how far critiques can reach. But what are these two "metanarratives" that Reed entrusts with an ultimate governing authority over a critical discourse? Before answering this question, I take a brief detour.

Central to what the appeal to postmodernism accomplishes in Reed's work is her view of science as consisting of paradigms. In American nursing science, paradigms are ubiquitous. In Reed's work, their place is pivotal. However, this omnipresence of paradigms both in nursing theory and nursing research has wide-reaching negative consequences for nursing scholarship, as critics pointed out (Paley, 2000a; Risjord, 2010). A critique of this obsolete view of science is an important thread in Risjord's (2010) analysis. Kuhn's work popularized the term *paradigm* far beyond the philosophy of science, with a perspective that science operates based on paradigms. One of the most lasting meanings of the term, as used by Kuhn, views paradigm as a "package" that encompasses philosophy, theories, and the corresponding methods. All components inside the paradigm cohere, but there is no coherence between the paradigms, that is, they are incommensurable. Post-Kuhnian philosophers pointed out debilitating limitations of a paradigm-based conception of science. In addition to representing an erroneous understanding of how science works, insulated paradigms imply the impossibility of criticism across them, which is a limitation for any intellectual field (Risjord, 2010).

Reed (1995) refers to the first "metanarrative" as *nursing philosophy* and uses this phrase interchangeably with two other notions, nursing worldviews and paradigms. Nurse scholars have articulated several "philosophic systems . . . such as . . . Parse's totality and simultaneity paradigms;[6] Newman's particulate-deterministic, interactive-integrative, and unitary-transformative worldviews; and Fawcett's reaction, reciprocal interaction, and simultaneous action worldviews" (Reed, 1995, p. 77). Medicine and psychology developed their respective paradigms too, as did other sciences, Reed claims. She then touches upon polarized positions in nursing literature about the desirability of such a paradigmatic diversity in nursing. While postmodernism eschews "the wholes and the unities" and while many authors support a paradigmatic diversity, Reed (1995) leans towards a preferred "metanarrative":

> The metanarrative of human developmental potential, transformational and self-transcendent capacity for health and healing, and recognition of the developmental histories of persons and their contexts. . . . [This view is] congruent with the philosophic ideas expressed in Newman's unitary-transformative paradigm and Parse's simultaneity paradigm.
>
> (p. 78)

This "nursing philosophy" then is a "metanarrative" that Reed (1995) puts forth as an expression of nursing's overarching values. We can recognize the influences from developmental psychology that inspired Reed's theory of self-transcendence, as well as her gesture to emphasize the congruence between these ideas and the selected extant nursing paradigms. As part of a new value-based neomodernist framework that presumably "incorporates both modernist and postmodernist philosophies" (p. 70), this "metanarrative of nursing philosophy" serves, in Reed's words, as "an external *corrective* of choice" (p. 78; italics added) for critiques of nursing science.[7] Although elsewhere Reed declares that "neomodernism champions an ongoing critique. . . [of] metanarratives" (2006b, p. 37), I suggest that setting "external correctives" for critique functions as a censorship and limits the scope and substance of criticism. At the same time, positioning the aforementioned expression of "nursing's values" as the "metanarrative" functioning as the *corrective* suggests that the assumptions underpinning the previous quote themselves safely escape postmodern contestations of, most notably, humanism, progress, and the metanarrative of (nursing) science.

Reed's (1995) discussion of the other "metanarrative," nursing practice, includes an affirmation of the link between science and practice in a way that moves beyond grand theorizing to advocate what she calls in her other publications "practice-based theory," an idea not uniformly accepted among nurse theorists. Reed appeals to postmodernism to support her focus on "practice": "In postmodernism, the ultimate locus of meaning is the culture or context of the object of inquiry" (p. 80). However, as in the previous example when the endorsement of criticism was cut short with a hasty comment that "critique alone is not enough," a tentative opening onto the "culture and context as something external to the person" (p. 80) is shut with a reminder that "the patient [is] a context of health and healing. Human beings' inner healing nature cannot be dismissed. . . . [The] patient [can be viewed] as environment" or as inseparably coexisting with it (p. 80). As I suggest in Chapters 6 and 7, recognition of "culture and context" – as agential in their own right, as preceding the individual, and as constituting social practices – is necessary to fully appreciate the nature of nursing practice. This is an insight from continentally informed nursing scholarship developed outside of the canon of American nursing theory by both non-American authors (e.g. Davina Allen, 2015; Latimer, 2003; May, 1990; Nelson, 2003; Purkis, 2003; Traynor, 2013) and a few American "outsiders" in the world of nursing theorising (e.g. David Allen, 1987; Drevdahl, 1999a, 1999b; Liaschenko, 1997; Sandelowski, 2003; Thompson, 1992). Reed's supposedly postmodern conception of "context," however, does not allow such an expanded appreciation of nursing practice to emerge.

In her discussion of the "metanarrative" of nursing practice, Reed (1995) contests a postmodern disinterest in "conceptualiz[ing] the whole" (p. 81) as a segue to reinstating the importance of nursing conceptual models. "The nursing conceptual models are a mechanism of translating the metanarrative of nursing practice for knowledge development" (pp. 80–81). We already encountered this idea when I delineated Reed's vision of practice-based theory, specifically, her proposal for conceptual resources "drawn in" to link with the "observations" from nurse–patient encounters. As I commented before, an account of practice, *translated* through extant nursing models and theories, constructs "practice" in a highly specific, limited, and some would suggest, problematic way (e.g. Drevdahl, 1999a; Latimer, 2003; May, 1990; Purkis, 1994, 1997, 2003). In Chapter 6 and other places, where I showcase early ground-breaking non-American postmodern and post-structural scholarship, I provide striking counter-examples of how these theoretical insights can inform understandings of nursing practice.

To recap my analysis of Reed's (1995) turn to postmodernism and beyond, to neomodernism, her attempt to transcend dichotomies in the name of postmodernism ironically reinforced some of the protracted binary oppositions in nursing: "traditional modern" science versus nursing science; social science paradigms versus nursing unique paradigms; and unitary-transformative nursing paradigm (for instance) versus other nursing paradigms. Next, the postmodern critical ethos is acknowledged only to be neutralized within the "neomodernist framework." "Metanarratives" in the form of nursing paradigms and extant conceptual models are explicitly re-affirmed. What is more, they are positioned beyond reproach, as the "external correctives to the critique of knowledge development" (p. 81). "Metanarratives" legitimize what counts as valid theory and critique in American nursing science and what can be seen/thought as nursing practice. Finally, despite a glimpse of "context" warranted by postmodernism, "environment" is inflected in Reed's version of nursing theory in such a way that the bottom line, the ultimate "phenomenon of concern to nursing" is "the patient's experience of health and healing" (p. 80). Although this nursing imperative is undeniable, the way this "phenomenon" is expressed in nursing theory and affirmed by Reed explicitly excludes the socially constructed nature of "experience" (e.g. the nurse–patient interaction as a social process occurring in a wider organizational and historical context) and at the same time assumes that a nurse has an unproblematic access to that "experience."

Reed's "neomodernism" dismisses inconvenient insights of postmodernism. The postmodern philosophy embedded within the intellectual matrix of American nursing science serves the maintenance function for the canonical conception of unique nursing knowledge and the pyramid view of nursing theory.

Jean Watson's "Postmodernism and Knowledge Development in Nursing," 1995

Another paper anthologized in Polifroni and Welch (1999), in addition to those by Dzurec (1989) and Reed (1995), is authored by Jean Watson, a Professor Emerita of nursing at the University of Colorado. Watson was named "one of the most prestigious nurse theorists of the 21st century" (Cox, 2000, p. 102). She founded the Caring Science Institute at her university and published prolifically from the late 1970s onwards. In her books, Watson elaborates, revises, and expands her vision of nursing as the science of caring, or human caring science. In the 1980s she postulated the ten carative factors, the first of which, for example, identifies the importance of "the formation of a humanistic-altruistic system of values" (Watson, 2005, p. 2). Watson (2012) describes her theoretical orientation as arising within a "phenomenological existential-spiritual realm"

(p. x). Commentaries on her work identify humanistic, existential, and transpersonal psychology as well as certain Indian and Chinese philosophies as the most important influences on her thinking (Sarter, 1988). Watson's Eastern-inspired belief in the inner self, or soul, as the most powerful source in human existence[8] (Sarter, 1988, p. 56) helps us place in context important notions in her work: the "unity of mind/body/spirit/nature/universe" tempered by the centrality of a "spirit-to-spirit connection" occurring within the "unitary field of consciousness" (e.g. Watson, 2005, p. 6).

Varied classifications of Watson's work reflect ongoing attempts in American nursing science to underscore the importance of formal properties of disciplinary theory. Thus, within Fawcett's (2005) structure of the disciplinary nursing knowledge, Watson's theory of human caring is placed alongside the works of Ida Jean Orlando and Hildegard Peplau as a middle-range theory. Textbooks surveying nursing theory (e.g. Alligood, 2014) categorize Watson's work as a "philosophy and theory of transpersonal caring." Watson's theory is said to belong to the human science tradition in nursing (Mitchell & Cody, 1992). These examples illustrate the paramount concern, within the American metatheoretical field, with the appropriate levelling and paradigmatic fit of theory.

Watson's metatheoretical comments provide yet another illustration of the kind and function of theory upheld within American nursing science. Caring science is proposed as the disciplinary foundation for the nursing profession (Watson, 2012). Nursing theories articulated within this science explicate "the ethical, philosophical, moral values, the world view, and lens one holds" (Watson, 2012, p. xi). Watson believes that metaphysical nursing systems nourish the profession: that her abstract writing on the ideal of caring can serve as a protective shield against the harsh realities of clinical nursing practice. She writes: "When things are so bad, we long for something else, for what might be, rather than succumb to what is" (Watson, 2005, p. xiii). The three interrelated themes listed here – nursing theory/philosophy as a foundation for the profession, as the ethical worldview, and as an ideal, timeless "core" transcending the "trim" of nursing realities (Watson, 2005, p. 3) – are common tropes in American nursing theoretical literature.

I now turn to examine Watson's ideas on postmodernism in her 1995 article, "Postmodernism and Knowledge Development in Nursing" and in the 1999 book *Postmodern Nursing and Beyond*. Watson's (1995) scope of bibliographic references is wider than Reed's (1995); that is, Watson cites Jacques Derrida, the semiotician responsible for "deconstruction"; Foucault; ground-breaking linguist, Ferdinand de Saussure; Lacanian psychoanalysis; founder of postcolonial studies Edward Said; and American feminist postmodernism scholar of education Patty Lather. Nevertheless, Watson's deployment of postmodernism and its implications for nursing science strikingly resemble those proposed by Reed.

At the outset, Watson (1995) equates the *modern* with "traditional, empiricist" science. She then emphasizes the crisis of modern science occasioned by certain postmodern ideas, which she links to nursing's human science paradigm. Watson's argument moves through three steps. She addresses the "shadow side of postmodernism: deconstruction" (p. 61), then moves "into the light of postmodernism: reconstruction" (p. 62), to ultimately rest in "nursing's most ancient and contemporary extant caring-healing-health knowledge and practices" (p. 63). In more concrete terms this means the following: The "shadow side" of postmodernism has precipitated "a void and moral confusion" (Watson, 1995, p. 20). The centre falls apart, leaving no epistemological and ethical foundations for nurses, a situation assessed by Watson as engendering rampant relativism. Thus, she concludes that the moral compass of nursing – contained in the work of the human science scholars Martha Rogers, Margaret Newman, Rosemarie Rizzo Parse, and her own – is needed more than ever. This precis shows how postmodern theory is employed by Watson to strengthen the position of a specific branch of "unique disciplinary knowledge," rather than to interrogate its foundations in the spirit of French theory.

Parts of Watson's writing can be described as poetic and metaphysical, for instance, when she invites "an awakening of human consciousness towards a deeper spiritual dimension of one's humanity" (Watson, 2005, p. 913), and this style is prominent in her 1999 book, *Postmodern Nursing and Beyond*. This work has been praised as moving, challenging, and spiritually inspiring (Cox, 2000), but not all commentators share such a view. Paley (2000b), appraising Watson's book for the discussion of postmodern ideas like the mistrust in metanarratives (the metanarratives of myth and religion as much as that of science), a questioning of Reason, the politics of difference, polyvocality, and the play of signifiers – which shook the academy in the 1990s – instead discovers a grandiose metanarrative of "new age nursing" (p. 82). Paley quickly realizes that in Watson's book, " 'postmodernism' is just a convenient, if totally inappropriate, peg on which to hang some unorthodox notions" (p. 82).[9] If these troubles created by postmodernism across the social science and humanities disciplines are not the centre of Watson's attention, then what does her evocation of "postmodernism" accomplish?

As in Reed's approach, the turn to postmodernism in Watson (1995, 1999) accomplishes the following ideological work: The structure of the article itself reinforces the idea of progress, of the movement from darkness to light; certain nursing paradigms and concepts (e.g. self-transcendence, holism) are valorized not only over "the traditional science" but also over other nursing paradigms and concepts (e.g. adaptation, linearity); and selected nursing theory is reinstated as a moral foundation for the profession. Cursorily acknowledging the postmodern challenges to dualisms, universal ethics, and metanarratives, Watson (1995) posits nursing science as an anti-Western-science metanarrative of "caring ethic" à la New Age (Paley, 2000b).

Following Reed's (1995) and Watson's (1995, 1999) "postmodern" writings, a new platitude has emerged in some textbooks on American nursing theory and nursing research (e.g. chapter by Clarke in B. Johnson & Webber, 2010; L. O. Walker & Avant, 2011): contrasting "modern," traditional, positivist, quantitative (read: backward) science with "postmodern," qualitative, subjectively orientated science/inquiry.

The prominence in American nursing theory literature of the anti-("traditional")-science sentiment reinvigorated by "postmodern" writings has provoked a reaction in defence of science *and* against French theory. "Postmodern nurse theorists," Glazer (2001) writes with derision, "are citing an impressive-sounding array of philosophers as supporting their abandonment of Western science" (p. 200). However, for a reader familiar with contemporary French theory, it is clear that Glazer's attack against postmodernism is misplaced: some nurse theorists' (e.g. Watson's) over-simplistic view of science is matched by their equally over-simplistic representation of postmodernism.[10] Equally, criticism of "postmodern ideas" by some Canadian scholars (e.g. Mackay, 2009; Stajduhar et al., 2001) in fact turn out to be directed not at this continental philosophical movement but at the extreme subjectivization and relativization of "truth" in American *nursing* grand theory. In other words, those Canadians attacked the caricature images of postmodernism found in some American nursing literature.

Nursing Science Quarterly

In 1988, Rosemarie Rizzo Parse, a prominent nurse theorist and the originator of the humanbecoming school of thought, then a professor of nursing at Hunter College in New York (later at Loyola University Chicago), opened the first issue of *Nursing Science Quarterly* (NSQ) by laying out the journal's intellectual boundaries: "It will focus on the publication of original works related to theory development, research, and practice, which *tie directly to the knowledge base as articulated in the extant nursing theories and frameworks*" (Parse, 1988, p. 1; italics added).

In keeping with its mandate, one of NSQ's primary achievements over the years has been promoting nursing as a basic (as opposed to "applied") science whose goal is to encourage discipline-specific theorizing. This positions NSQ as the voice *par excellence* (to use Risjord's vocabulary) in the consensus discourse of nursing theory in the United States. An attitude towards "borrowed theory" upheld within this conception of nursing science is outlined in the previous chapter. Perhaps the clearest expression of this highly negative attitude can be found in William Cody's (1998) response to some nurses' growing interest in interdisciplinary "discourses from orthodox Marxism to radical feminism" (p. 44). One of Cody's objections to "critical theory" as a guide of nursing practice rests in the absence of nurses' effort to connect critical theory borrowed from sociology to extant nursing frameworks. Quite predictably, over more than two decades, references in NSQ to ("borrowed") postmodern and post-structural theory and Foucault's work can be counted on the fingers of one hand.

What are the discursive conditions of possibility that enable (partial) recognition of postmodernism, post-structuralism, and Foucault in NSQ? How were postmodernism and post-structuralism "packaged" in order to gain acceptance onto the pages of this journal? We have already encountered Watson's "Postmodernism and Knowledge Development in Nursing" published in NSQ in 1995. This version of "postmodernism" avoids any critical engagement with binaries, metanarratives, and politics of difference and serves to reaffirm the "cosmic caring" metanarrative of (Watson's vision of) the nursing's human science tradition. Other references to postmodernism and Foucault in NSQ, described in the following, are equally entangled within the conception of unique science and discipline-specific theory.

Topaz et al. (2014) conceive of postmodernism as an evolutionary stage in the process of metatheoretical development (à la Reed, 1995), which is subsumed by the next, developmentally superior stage. Topaz et al. follow this trope when presenting a middle-range nursing theory of successful aging, called *gerotranscendence*, which, according to the authors, replaces weakness-based, functionalist theories of aging de-centred in the wake of postmodern critiques of ageism. (What makes the theory of gerotranscendence a *nursing* theory is "derivation" of some components of this theory from Roy's adaptation model.) Similar to my point in relation to Reed's article, Topaz et al.'s evolutionary reading of postmodernism as a mere stage effectively positions their theory as if outside of (postmodern) questioning of the contemporary societal discourses constructing the discourse of "successful aging" itself as an ideal (O'Rourke & Ceci, 2013).

In another article in NSQ, titled "Power, Right, and Truth: Foucault's Triangle as a Model for Clinical Power," Polifroni (2010) proposes "a model of power . . . consistent with the worldview in the 21st century for nursing practice" (p. 8). Polifroni, operating under a similarly limited understanding of the *nursingness* of nursing theory, embeds Foucault's notion of power within two conceptualizations of power by nurses: Peggy Chinn's PEACE framework (Praxis, Empowerment, Awareness, Cooperation, and Evolvement) and Elizabeth Barrett's nursing theory of *power of*. According to Barrett, power is "the capacity to participate knowingly in the nature of change characterizing the continuous patterning of the human and environmental fields" (Caroselli & Barrett, 1998, cited in Polifroni, 2010, p. 11). Foucault's notion of power is imagined by Polifroni as a "triangle of power, right, and truth": "If power is everywhere and it is inextricably connected to knowledge and truth, which are essential rights for all, then all individuals have power" (p. 11). Combining Chinn's, Barrett's, and Foucault's "conceptualizations," Polifroni proposes a model of clinical power for nurses. "Picture two triangles – the outer, . . . with power at the base and right and truth on each arm, within which is a second triangle called *clinical power*, with relationship and awareness on its arms" (Polifroni, 2010, p. 12). "Power [in Foucault] becomes emancipatory as knowledge and truth are discovered and disseminated" (Polifroni, 2010, p. 11).

This example vividly illustrates how nurse authors transform "borrowed" ideas into "discipline-specific" models. If anything at all can be said about such a strange exercise, it is that an outcome of these mental gymnastics is the stripping of Foucault's ideas of their meaning: Contradicting his capillary image of power, certain kinds of relationships and situations (presumably, an ideal nurse–patient interaction) are hailed as fundamentally and unquestioningly benevolent arrangements – such as relationships built on "love and not dominance" (Polifroni, 2010, p. 10). This is a stark misrepresentation of Foucault: The power/

knowledge nexus is transformed into a claim that more knowledge equals more power in Polifroni's liberal humanist rendition.

Ironically, I found only one instance when "continental philosophy" and Foucault are granted full autonomy in *NSQ*. Mitchell and Cody (2002) discuss the hostility with which the human science nursing tradition has been met in mainstream nursing and contrast it with the welcoming recognition of what they describe as human science continental philosophers like Heidegger, Gadamer, and Foucault in other disciplines in the American academy. Thus, my exposition of the applications of postmodernism, post-structuralism, and Foucault in *NSQ* has come full circle: I started with Cody's (1998) uncompromising position towards "borrowed theory," a position requiring that in order to become useful, borrowed ideas should undergo a conceptual transformation in the fire of "extant nursing theory" (as illustrated in Topaz et al. and Polifroni). And I concluded with Mitchel and Cody's (2002) clear demarcation of Foucault's "proper" place *outside* of nursing's disciplinary pyramid.

Concluding Thoughts

In this chapter, I started examining deployments of postmodern and post-structural theory in American nursing theory literature. Gortner, a "traditional" nurse scientist, dismissed Foucault as a "philosopher of the month": one of those philosophical imposters attempting to relativize the legitimacy of scientific truth (Gortner, 1993/1997). Gortner's objection to continental philosophical schools presented in American nursing literature as alternative *scientific* paradigms, however, invites the following observation, which surprisingly has not been seriously attended to in nursing: Nurses persistently claim scientific status for the kinds of scholarship that are better understood as humanities-type inquiry and theorizing, a conception that can facilitate useful interdisciplinary dialogues and enrich the discipline of nursing (see also C. Holmes, 1991; Thompson, 1985).

The humanbecoming scholars expressed if not an outright rejection of Foucault and other critical theory, then a firm placement of Foucault outside of unique nursing knowledge (Mitchell & Cody, 2002). Foucault and other continental philosophers exemplify "borrowed theory": useful, but "other." To transform borrowed theory into proper nursing scholarship, nurse authors (e.g. Polifroni, 2010) have undertaken a "reformulation," linking Foucault's "conceptions" with the "extant nursing theories and frameworks."

As I discussed in the previous chapter, an understanding of the relationship between *theory* and *concept* displayed in such "reformulation" or "derivation" approaches has been criticized (Paley, 2006; Risjord, 2010). These approaches are one of the clearest contemporary incarnations of the logical positivist understanding of language and theory. The end result of such intellectual projects is the stripping of continental ideas of their specific, context-bound meanings.

Those American nurse theorists who engaged with postmodern and post-structural ideas have thoroughly assimilated them within their respective well-established theories and "worldviews." The process of assimilation has taken two predominant forms: selectivity and addition, explained in the following. Often-cited and anthologized work by Watson (1995) and Reed (1995) embraced aspects of postmodernism (i.e. selectivity), allowing an ongoing rejection of the metanarrative of medical science. However, no parallel interrogation of the (metanarrative of) unique nursing knowledge occurred. Moreover, the latter was rhetorically repositioned at the higher evolutionary level (called *neomodernism* or *caring science*) transcending "postmodern criticisms."

The other form of assimilation was done by addition. A plurality was proposed whereby no theory, approach, paradigm, or method need be rejected (Dzurec, 1989). This view of knowledge development seems to be widely shared in the discipline of nursing. Indeed, recognition of intellectual diversity is a hallmark of academic nursing, serving the discipline well. When this can become prob-lematic, as sometimes happens in nursing literature, is when the notion of incompatible paradigms of science is deployed to seal off "coherent packages of philosophy-theory-methods" from "outside" criticism.

Notes

1   I underline these words to emphasize the degree to which the field of American nurs-ing *theory* is coterminous with the notion of science, as opposed to, say, the humani-ties. Our everyday use makes these journal titles so familiar that we do not question what is meant by the term "science" in American theoretical discourse and what this linkage of nursing theory with science enables or proscribes.

2   This ostensible requirement of compatibility owes to the entrenched notion of para-digms, extracted from Kuhn's writings, and remains in nursing despite critiques of *paradigm* in the philosophy of science. Interestingly, Gortner's writings prefigure more recent critiques (e.g. Paley, 2000a; Risjord, 2010) of the entrenched paradigmatic thinking and its attendant requirement of coherence among a researcher's philosophy, ontology, and methods.

3   Admittedly, Gortner's depiction of science does not seem to acknowledge feminist criticisms of science like those presented by Sandra Harding (1986/1999, 1995). Instead, Gortner focuses on *nursing* papers in *Advances in Nursing Science* that intro-duced feminist ideas into nursing in the 1980s. This American feminist nursing lit-erature tends to draw eclectically on various strands of feminist theory often without making important distinctions among them. I believe that Harding's and other sci-entists' (e.g. Haraway, Dorothy Smith, Heckman) robust feminist critiques of science must accompany readings in philosophy of science in nursing programs. This lack of acknowledgement of feminist critiques of science by Gortner, however, does not invalidate her appraisal of "alternative scientific methods" in nursing.

4   Later, Parse capitalized the lower case "h" of humanbecoming; however, my lower case "h" reflects the usage in my cited material.

5   Reed is not explicit about how this process of practice-based theorizing would look. The notion of a corrective that I introduced here is discussed further in the chapter. Reed does not provide any examples of the external corrective, but her formulation of the "metanarrative" seems to be devised with such a purpose in mind. American nursing theories, including those singled out by Reed as suitable "correctives" for nurs-ing theorizing, treat sociological concepts in a colloquial way, if at all (Kim & Kollak, 2006). Thus, problematically, any empirical "social facts" and conceptualizations of nursing practice enabled by contemporary *social theory* simply fall outside of (Reed's) vision enabled by the "nursing-specific spectacles."

6 Nurse theorist Parse, the author of humanbecoming theory, who previously put forth these two paradigms (her own theory fell within the simultaneity paradigm), later set her theory as a separate, third entity: humanbecoming paradigm (Cody, 2015).

7 Reed is not explicit about how this "corrective" is supposed to work. As I understand it, nursing's metanarrative in the form of selected grand theories is proposed by Reed as legitimating what criticisms of nursing ideas can be accepted and what should be rejected as compromising nursing's "foundational" ideas/ideals. I interpret Reed's recourse to neomodernism as an attempt to safeguard the established body of American nursing theory.

8 Watson's use of Eastern philosophies appears to be superficial and limited to use of images and symbols on her website that allude to ancient Eastern philosophies and religions, but do not represent their belief systems with depth or accuracy. For example, the lotus (Buddhist thought) is used as the Watson Caring Science Institute logo, and various items for sale on the website suggest a trivialization of ancient Eastern philosophies and religions: a crystal charm in the shape of Buddha for the "Caritas" charm bracelet, a seven-Chakras (Hinduism) gemstone bracelet, and a Yin-Yang (ancient Chinese philosophy) gold bead charm.

9 Paley's (2000b) critique is far from bashing Watson's (1999) ideas wholesale. Rather, he points out the book's undiscriminating mixture of ideas and a complete avoidance of the reputable academic sources that can actually *support* some of Watson's claims.

10 Thompson (2002) correctly points out Glazer's (2001) mistaken generalization that all postmodern nursing scholarship is lacking in rigour.

References

Allen, D. G. (1987). The social policy statement: A reappraisal. *Advances in Nursing Science*, 10(1), 39–48.

Allen, D. G. (2015). *The invisible work of nurses: Hospitals, organisation and healthcare*. Routledge.

Alligood, M. R. (Ed.). (2014). *Nursing theorists and their work* (8th ed.). Mosby Elsevier.

Alligood, M. R. (Ed.). (2018). *Nursing theorists and their work* (9th ed.). Elsevier.

Alligood, M. R., & Tomey, A. M. (Eds.). (2010). *Nursing theorists and their work* (7th ed.). Mosby Elsevier.

Chinn, P. L., & Kramer, M. K. (2004). *Integrated knowledge development in nursing* (6th ed.). Mosby.

Chinn, P. L., & Kramer, M. K. (2008). *Integrated theory and knowledge development in nursing* (7th ed.). Mosby Elsevier.

Chinn, P. L., & Kramer, M. K. (2011). *Integrated theory and knowledge development in nursing* (8th ed.). Elsevier Mosby.

Chinn, P. L., & Kramer, M. K. (2015). *Knowledge development in nursing: Theory and process* (9th ed.). Elsevier Health Sciences.

Chinn, P. L., & Kramer, M. K. (2019). *Knowledge development in nursing: Theory and process* (10th ed.). Mosby Elsevier.

Cody, W. K. (1998). Critical theory and nursing science: Freedom in theory and practice. *Nursing Science Quarterly*, 11(2), 44–46.

Cody, W. K. (Ed.). (2006). *Philosophical and theoretical perspectives for advanced nursing practice* (4th ed.). Jones and Bartlett Publishers.

Cody, W. K. (2015). Book review. The humanbecoming paradigm: A transformational worldview. *Nursing Science Quarterly*, 28(2), 172–173.

Cox, C. L. (2000). Book review: Postmodern nursing and beyond by Jean Watson. *Complementary Therapies in Clinical Practice, 6*(2), 102.

Drevdahl, D. (1999a). Sailing beyond: Nursing theory and the person. *Advances in Nursing Science, 21*(4), 1–13.

Drevdahl, D. (1999b). Meanings of community in a community health center. *Public Health Nursing, 16*(6), 417–425.

Dzurec, L. (1989). The necessity for and evolution of multiple paradigms for nursing research: A poststructuralist perspective. *Advances in Nursing Science, 11*(4), 69–77.

Fawcett, J. (2005). *Contemporary nursing knowledge: Analysis and evaluation of nursing models and theories* (2nd ed.). F. A. Davis.

Fitzpatrick, J. J., & McCarthy, G. (Eds). (2014). *Theories guiding nursing research and practice: Making nursing knowledge development explicit.* Springer Publishing Company.

Fitzpatrick, J. J., & Whall, A. L. (2005). *Conceptual models of nursing: Analysis and application* (4th ed.). Pearson.

Fitzpatrick, J. J., & Whall, A. L. (Eds.). (2016). *Conceptual models of nursing: Global perspectives* (5th ed.). Pearson.

Glazer, S. (2001). Therapeutic touch and postmodernism in nursing. *Nursing Philosophy, 2*(3), 196–212.

Gortner, S. R. (1991). Historical development of doctoral programs: Shaping our expectations. *Journal of Professional Nursing, 7*(1), 45–53.

Gortner, S. R. (1997a). Nursing science in transition. In L. H. Nicoll (Ed.), *Perspectives on nursing theory* (3rd ed., pp. 265–271). Lippincott. (Original work published in *Nursing Research, 29*(3), 180–183, in 1980)

Gortner, S. R. (1997b). Nursing values and science: Toward a science philosophy. In L. H. Nicoll (Ed.), *Perspectives on nursing theory* (3rd ed., pp. 197–206). Lippincott. (Original work published in *Image: Journal of Nursing Scholarship, 22*(2), 101–105, in 1990)

Gortner, S. R. (1997c). Nursing's syntax revisited: A critique of philosophies said to influence nursing theories. In L. H. Nicoll (Ed.), *Perspectives on nursing theory* (3rd ed., pp. 357–368). Lippincott. (Original work published in *International Journal of Nursing Studies, 30*(6), 477–488, in 1993)

Gortner, S. R. (1997d). Research for a practice profession. In L. H. Nicoll (Ed.), *Perspectives on nursing theory* (3rd ed., pp. 693–700). Lippincott. (Original work published in *Nursing Research, 24*(3), 193–197, in 1975)

Gortner, S. R. (1997e). The history and philosophy of nursing science and research. In L. H. Nicoll (Ed.), *Perspectives on nursing theory* (3rd ed., pp. 286–292). Lippincott. (Original work published in *Advances in Nursing Science, 5*(2), 1–8, in 1983)

Gortner, S. R. (2000). Knowledge development in nursing: Our historical roots and future opportunities. *Nursing Outlook, 48*(2), 60–67.

Harding, S. (1995). The method question. In A. Omery, C. E. Kasper, & G. G. Page (Eds.), *In search of nursing science* (pp. 106–126). SAGE.

Harding, S. (1999). The instability of the analytical categories of feminist theory. In E. C. Polifroni & M. Welch (Eds.), *Perspectives on philosophy of science in nursing: An historical and contemporary anthology* (pp. 396–410). Lippincott Williams & Wilkins. (Original work published in *Signs, 11*(4), 645–664, in 1986)

Holmes, C. A. (1991). Theory: Where are we going and what have we missed along the way? In G. Gray & R. Pratt (Eds.), *Towards a discipline of nursing* (pp. 435–460). Churchill Livingstone.

Johnson, B. M., & Webber, P. B. (2010). *An introduction to theory and reasoning in nursing* (3rd ed.). Lippincott Williams & Wilkins.

Kenney, J. W. (Ed.). (1996). *Philosophical and theoretical perspectives for advanced nursing practice*. Jones and Bartlett Publishers.

Kenney, J. W. (Ed.). (2002). *Philosophical and theoretical perspectives for advanced nursing practice* (3rd ed.). Jones and Bartlett Publishers.

Kim, H. S., & Kollak, I. (Eds.). (2006). *Nursing theories: Conceptual and philosophical foundations* (2nd ed.). Springer Publishing Company.

Latimer, J. (2003). *Advanced qualitative research for nursing*. Blackwell Science Ltd.

Letourneau, N., & Allen, M. (1999). Post-positivistic critical multiplism: A beginning dialogue. *Journal of Advanced Nursing, 30*(3), 623–630.

Liaschenko, J. (1997). Ethics and the geography of the nurse–patient relationship: Spatial vulnerabilities and gendered space. *Scholarly Inquiry for Nursing Practice, 11*(1), 45–59.

Mackay, M. (2009). Why nursing has not embraced the clinician-scientist role. *Nursing Philosophy, 10*(4), 287–296.

May, C. (1990). Research on nurse–patient relationships: Problems of theory, problems of practice. *Journal of Advanced Nursing, 15*(3), 307–315.

Meleis, A. I. (1997). *Theoretical nursing: Development and progress* (3rd ed.). Lippincott.

Meleis, A. I. (2007). *Theoretical nursing: Development and progress* (4th ed.). Lippincott Williams & Wilkins.

Meleis, A. I. (2012). *Theoretical nursing: Development and progress* (5th ed.). Wolters Kluwer/Lippincott Williams & Wilkins.

Mitchell, G. J., & Bournes, D. A. (2006). Challenging the atheoretical production of nursing knowledge: A response to Reed and Rolfe's column. *Nursing Science Quarterly, 19*(2), 116–119.

Mitchell, G. J., & Cody, W. K. (1992). Nursing knowledge and human science: Ontological and epistemological considerations. *Nursing Science Quarterly, 5*, 54–61.

Mitchell, G. J., & Cody, W. K. (2002). Ambiguous opportunity: Toiling for truth of nursing art and science. *Nursing Science Quarterly, 15*, 71–79.

Munhall, P. L. (1982). Nursing philosophy and nursing research: In apposition or opposition? *Nursing Research, 31*(3), 176–177, 181.

Nelson, S. (2003). A history of small things. In J. Latimer (Ed.), *Advanced qualitative research for nursing* (pp. 211–230). Blackwell Science Ltd.

Nicoll, L. H. (Ed.). (1997). *Perspectives on nursing theory* (3rd ed.). Lippincott.

Omery, A., Kasper, C. E., & Page, G. (Eds.). (1995). *In search of nursing science*. SAGE.

O'Rourke, H. M., & Ceci, C. (2013). Reexamining the boundaries of the "normal" in ageing. *Nursing Inquiry, 20*(1), 51–59.

Packard, S. A., & Polifroni, E. C. (1999). The dilemma of nursing science: Current quandaries and lack of direction. In E. C. Polifroni & M. Welch (Eds.), *Perspectives on philosophy of science in nursing: An historical and contemporary anthology* (pp. 498–506). Lippincott Williams & Wilkins. (Original work published in *Nursing Science Quarterly, 4*(1), 7–13, in 1991)

Paley, J. (2000a). Paradigms and presuppositions: The difference between qualitative and quantitative research. *Scholarly Inquiry for Nursing Practice, 14*(2), 143–155.

Paley, J. (2000b). Book review: Postmodern nursing and beyond. *Nursing Philosophy, 1*(1), 82–83.

Paley, J. (2002). Caring as a slave morality: Nietzschean themes in nursing. *Journal of Advanced Nursing, 40*(1), 25–35.

Paley, J. (2006). Book review: Nursing theorists and their work. *Nursing Philosophy, 7*(4), 275–280.

Parker, M. E. (2006). *Nursing theories and nursing practice* (2nd ed.). F. A. Davis.

Parker, M. E., & Smith, M. C. (2010). *Nursing theories and nursing practice* (3rd ed.). F. A. Davis.

Parse, R. R. (1988). Beginnings. *Nursing Science Quarterly, 1*(1), 1–2.

Polifroni, E. C. (2010). Power, right, and truth: Foucault's triangle as a model for clinical power. *Nursing Science Quarterly, 23*(1), 8–12.

Polifroni, E. C., & Welch, M. (Eds.). (1999). *Perspectives on philosophy of science in nursing: An historical and contemporary anthology.* Lippincott Williams & Wilkins.

Purkis, M. E. (1994). Entering the field: Intrusions of the social and its exclusion from studies of nursing practice. *International Journal of Nursing Studies, 31*(4), 315–336.

Purkis, M. E. (1997). The "social determinants" of practice? A critical analysis of the discourse of health promotion. *The Canadian Journal of Nursing Research, 29*(1), 47–62.

Purkis, M. E. (2003). Moving nursing practice: Integrating theory and method. In J. Latimer (Ed.), *Advanced qualitative research for nursing* (pp. 32–50). Blackwell Science Ltd.

Reed, P. G. (1991). Toward a nursing theory of self-transcendence: Deductive reformulation using developmental theories. *Advances in Nursing Science, 13*(4), 64–77.

Reed, P. G. (1995). A treatise on nursing knowledge development for the 21st century: Beyond postmodernism. *Advances in Nursing Science, 17*(3), 70–84.

Reed, P. G. (1996). Transforming practice knowledge into nursing knowledge – a revisionist analysis of Peplau. *Journal of Nursing Scholarship, 28*(1), 29–33.

Reed, P. G. (2000). Nursing reformation: Historical reflections and philosophic foundations. *Nursing Science Quarterly, 13*(2), 129–136.

Reed, P. G. (2006a). The practice turn in nursing epistemology. *Nursing Science Quarterly, 19*(1), 36–38.

Reed, P. G. (2006b). Commentary on neomodernism and evidence-based nursing: Implications for the production of nursing knowledge. *Nursing Outlook, 54*(1), 36–38.

Reed, P. G. (2008). Practitioner as theorist: A reprise. *Nursing Science Quarterly, 21*(4), 315–321.

Reed, P. G., & Shearer, N. B. C. (2009). *Perspectives on nursing theory* (5th ed.). Wolters Kluwer/Lippincott Williams & Wilkins.

Reed, P. G., & Shearer, N. B. C. (2012). *Perspectives on nursing theory* (6th ed.). Wolters Kluwer/Lippincott Williams & Wilkins.

Risjord, M. (2010). *Nursing knowledge: Science, practice, and philosophy.* Wiley-Blackwell.

Roy, C., Sr., & Jones, D. A. (Eds.). (2007). *Nursing knowledge development and clinical practice.* Springer Publishing Company.

Sandelowski, M. (2003). Taking things seriously: Studying the material culture of nursing. In J. Latimer (Ed.), *Advanced qualitative research for nursing* (pp. 185–210). Blackwell Science Ltd.

Sarter, B. (1988). Philosophical sources of nursing theory. *Nursing Science Quarterly, 1*(2), 52–59.

Schumacher, K. L., & Gortner, S. R. (1992). (Mis)conceptions and reconceptions about traditional science. *Advances in Nursing Science, 14*, 1–11.

Silva, M. C., & Rothbart, D. (1997). An analysis of changing trends in philosophies of science on nursing theory development and testing. In L. H. Nicoll (Ed.), *Perspectives on nursing theory* (3rd ed., pp. 293–306). Lippincott. (Original work published in *Advances in Nursing Science, 6*(2), 1–13, in 1984)

Smith, M. J., & Liehr, P. R. (Eds.). (2014). *Middle range theory for nursing* (3rd ed.). Springer.

Stajduhar, K. I., Balneaves, L., & Thorne, S. E. (2001). A case for the "middle ground": Exploring the tensions of postmodern thought in nursing. *Nursing Philosophy, 2*(1), 72–82.

Thompson, J. L. (1985). Practical discourse in nursing: Going beyond empiricism and historicism. *Advances in Nursing Science, 7*(4), 59–71.

Thompson, J. L. (1992). Identity politics, essentialism, and constructions of "home" in nursing. In J. L. Thompson, D. G. Allen, & L. Rodriguez-Fisher (Eds.), *Critique, resistance, and action: Working papers in the politics of nursing* (pp. 21–34). NLN.

Thompson, J. L. (2002). Which postmodernism? A critical response to therapeutic touch and postmodernism in nursing. *Nursing Philosophy, 3*(1), 58–62.

Thorne, S. E., Canam, C., Dahinten, S., Hall, W., Henderson, A., & Kirkham, S. R. (1998). Nursing's metaparadigm concepts: Disimpacting the debates. *Journal of Advanced Nursing, 27*(6), 1257–1268.

Thorne, S. E., Henderson, A. D., McPherson, G. I., & Pesut, B. K. (2004). The problematic allure of the binary in nursing theoretical discourse. *Nursing Philosophy, 5*(3), 208–215.

Tomey, A. M., & Alligood, M. R. (Eds.). (1998). *Nursing theorists and their work* (4th ed.). Mosby.

Tomey, A. M., & Alligood, M. R. (Eds.). (2002). *Nursing theorists and their work* (5th ed.). Mosby Elsevier.

Tomey, A. M., & Alligood, M. R. (Eds.). (2006). *Nursing theorists and their work* (6th ed.). Mosby.

Topaz, M., Troutman-Jordan, M., & MacKenzie, M. (2014). Construction, deconstruction, and reconstruction: The roots of successful aging theories. *Nursing Science Quarterly, 27*(3), 226–233.

Traynor, M. (2013). *Nursing in context: Policy, politics, profession.* Palgrave Macmillan.

Walker, L. O., & Avant, K. C. (2005). *Strategies for theory construction in nursing* (4th ed.). Pearson Prentice Hall.

Walker, L. O., & Avant, K. C. (2011). *Strategies for theory construction in nursing* (5th ed.). Pearson Prentice Hall.

Watson, J. (1995). Postmodernism and knowledge development in nursing. *Nursing Science Quarterly, 8*(2), 60–64.

Watson, J. (1999). *Postmodern nursing and beyond.* Churchill Livingstone.

Watson, J. (2005). *Caring science as sacred science.* F. A. Davis.

Watson, J. (2012). *Human caring science: A theory of nursing* (2nd ed.). Jones and Bartlett Learning.

5 Postmodern and Post-Structural Ideas in American Nursing Texts II

Advances in Nursing Science and the Enclave Group

In this chapter, I continue my exploration of American nursing scholarship published from the late 1980s throughout the first decade of the 2000s that claims to draw on postmodern and post-structural concepts. The primary focus in this chapter is *Advances in Nursing Science* (*ANS*), a journal well respected for its broad theoretical scope and critical orientation. It is in this journal that we encounter (in the American context) a diversity of papers informed by French theory and American feminist writings. However, as I illustrate in this chapter, despite *ANS*'s openness to continental philosophy and interdisciplinary theory, this journal had developed a narrative, nursing as emancipatory practice, which shaped what kinds of continental philosophy were usually discussed on the pages of *ANS* and how philosophical ideas including post-structural were applied. Thus, I point out the continuity of this chapter with the previous chapter. That is, the majority of publications in *ANS* referred to in this chapter exhibit patterns similar to those identified in the preceding chapter: superficial reading of postmodern and post-structural theory and enduring attempts (manifesting to various degrees) to reconcile French theory with the two overarching agendas: (a) the perpetuation of the metatheoretical nursing discourse that reveals implicit or explicit assumptions of the American nursing theory matrix and (b) the contribution to the discourse of "emancipatory nursing."

In this chapter I also showcase the work of a loosely connected group of American nurse scholars writing on the margins of American nursing theory (and not being its proponents), whom I call the *enclave group*, distinguished by their insightful applications of continental philosophy. Publications by the enclave scholars in *ANS* and other nursing journals employed postmodern and post-structural ideas in a well-informed way that differed markedly from the use of French theory in American nursing theoretical writings examined thus far. Significantly, the enclave scholars critically engaged with American nursing science/theory (e.g. by contributing chapters to selected edited volumes) while proposing alternative theoretical directions for nursing scholarship. These writings, however, have not become part of a widely circulated canon of "nursing knowledge/nursing theory" textbooks. (Refer to Tables A1 and A2 for a list of American nursing literature that claims postmodern and post-structural influences.) Thus, this chapter continues an examination of American nursing postmodern and

DOI: 10.4324/9781003194439-5

post-structural scholarship to deepen our awareness of the profound influence of the conception of "unique nursing knowledge/nursing theory" on the intelligibility of interdisciplinary theory. The American nursing disciplinary matrix continually produced unintelligibility of the most radical (and thus offering great potential for a re-examination of sedimented views) French theoretical anti-humanist ideas and other social theory not amenable to the discourses of "nursing science" and "emancipatory practice."[1]

As in the previous chapter, I begin with providing relevant context about the ANS journal and its editor, Peggy Chinn, whose unwavering leadership influenced American nursing science in distinctive ways. What might seem like a long lead-up to a discussion of postmodern and post-structural scholarship in ANS is meant to expand our understanding of the American theoretical nursing scene.

Postmodern and Post-structural Theory in *Advances in Nursing Science*

The Journal

In 1978, three nursing journals were launched in the United States: *Advances in Nursing Science* (ANS; with a broad theoretical mandate), *Western Journal of Nursing Research*, and *Research in Nursing and Health*. As discussed previously, in the late 1970s, *theoretical* discourse in the discipline had been firmly positioned as a "nursing science" project. Worth noticing is the demarcation of this latter domain of "nursing science" from that of "nursing research" (i.e. of a kind deemed suitable for nursing *research* journals). It is still a largely unexplored question in nursing of how these historical divisions have contributed to the understandings of the notion of theory and the guises and uses of theory in science, research, and scholarship in the discipline.

Since its inception, ANS has prospered under the editorship of Peggy Chinn, then professor of nursing at Wright State University in Ohio and presently Professor Emerita, University of Connecticut. When one leafs through the ANS archives, it becomes clear that the topics and directions set out in its first issue, titled "Practice-Oriented Theory," have influenced the journal's long history. Alluding to the prevailing theoretical discourse in nursing about levels of theory, the inaugural issue identified the journal's focus on practical applications of nursing models, on the derivation of "practice-level" theories from the more abstract ones, and on the formulation of theories that remain close to the world of nursing practice (as opposed to grand theories). This focus challenged the understanding of nursing as a *basic* science (e.g. J. Johnson, 1991), while still maintaining a sympathetic eye on nursing theories and promoting metatheoretical discussions.

The first issue of ANS included Jacqueline Fawcett's (1978/1997) paper "The Relationship between Theory and Research: A Double Helix." As I have indicated in Chapter 3, Fawcett's articulation of the structure of scientific theory, concepts, and conceptual models is possibly the most illustrative manifestation of the logical positivist influence on the nursing discipline. Further, her vision of proper discipline-specific research as "directed to one of two goals – theory building or theory testing" where *theory* refers exclusively to nursing-specific theory (Fawcett, 1978/1997, p. 720) – solidifies a line separating "nursing science" focused on the discipline-specific theory/research from *other* nursing research, for example, housed in the two American research journals named earlier. Fawcett's paper in the premiere issue of *ANS* has undoubtedly contributed to the lasting influence of these ideas.

Another article in the first issue of *ANS*, Barbara Carper's (1978) "Fundamental Patterns of Knowing in Nursing," famously delineated "empirics, aesthetics, ethics, and personal knowing" as distinctive yet overlapping ways in which nurses *know*. The influence of this publication on broader nursing scholarship is difficult to overestimate; its fortunate, perhaps strategic, placement at the forefront of a leading American theoretical nursing journal ensured that the four original patterns of knowing and their subsequent extension (e.g. Chinn & Kramer, 2008, 2011; Jacobs-Kramer & Chinn, 1988/1997; White, 1995) have steered the journal's course of advancing nursing science. Many authors have situated their own thinking within one or another "pattern." Laying out four diverse patterns of knowing as a foundation for ensuing academic discussions has allowed *ANS* to promote an image of inclusive and integrative nursing science. For instance, the journal devoted separate thematic issues to nursing diagnosis, nursing intervention, and "physiological variables" – topics rejected in some nursing quarters for mimicking medicine. *ANS* addressed with equal interest "ethics and values" and philosophy of science; holistic health and nursing informatics; and quantitative research and phenomenological research (e.g. Benner, 1985), among other topics. It is noteworthy that Chinn also extended and modified the four original patterns of knowing into a framework for her well-known co-authored book on nursing knowledge development and evaluation (e.g. Chinn & Kramer, 2004).[2]

In addition to an image of *integrative* science built upon diverse ways of knowing and focused on practice-oriented theories, nursing science emerged in *ANS* as having a high regard for "models" and "frameworks," albeit not of a grand type. In other words, there were preferred rhetorical strategies or specific ways to talk about nursing science employed across many publications in *ANS*. These linguistic preferences reflect a belief about the desired goals of theoretical activity in the discipline of nursing – ideally, the goal is creation of formal(ized) models that can be given a theorist's name and then, for instance, deployed to guide curricular and organizational designs or approaches to care delivery. Thus, in the first issue of the journal, Chinn and Jacobs (1978) proposed a *model* for theory development in nursing. The importance of formal(ized) models and formal theorizing has been consistently emphasized by Chinn elsewhere (Kagan & Chinn, 2010; Kagan et al., 2014, p. 3).

I suggest that one effect of such an emphasis on "frameworks" and "models" (a conception of "model" commonly assumed in *ANS* is discussed in endnote 11 to Chapter 3) is the codification of specific textual or knowledge-construction practices that privilege a clear identification of theory or methodology that is announced in the article's title. The latter approach is seen at work in many

ANS publications, as can be gleaned from the following examples: "The Quality-Caring Model©: Blending Dual Paradigms" (Duffy & Hoskins, 2003) or "Reconceptualizing Vulnerability: Deconstruction and Reconstruction as a Postmodern Feminist Analytical Research Method" (Glass & Davis, 2004). These titles signal their belonging to the discourse of "nursing knowledge" by mobilizing the American disciplinary jargon of paradigms (in the former example) and of a composite methodological orientation where "deconstruction" is (compulsorily) balanced with "reconstruction" as a positive end-point of analysis (in the latter). This codification of particular kinds of linguistic tropes reinforces what counts as legitimate theoretical discourse in the discipline.

A feature of ANS, positioning it apart from a narrow vision of a "unique" discipline cautious towards borrowed theory, was that ANS welcomed publications based on interdisciplinary theory.[3] Particularly noticeable in the 1990s and early 2000s were the two theoretical leanings of the journal – feminist and critical theory – which seemed to parallel explicit life-long values of Chinn, the journal's editor. It was not accidental that the first issue of ANS featured an article by Jo Ann Ashley, then professor of nursing at Wright State University in Ohio. Chinn later identified Ashley as her teacher and a noted feminist, and she often cited Ashley's book, *Hospitals, Paternalism, and the Role of the Nurse* (1976). This book is "a critique of a patriarchally defined medical system that systematically exploits women as patients, wives, and nurses" (Chinn, 1995, p. 274). In the early 1980s Chinn co-founded a Radical Feminist Nurses Network, Cassandra, described as a voice of struggle for equal rights for women (Chinn, n.d., "Projects" tab, "Cassandra"). This version of feminism "values and endorses women, critiques male thinking, challenges patriarchal systems, and focuses on creating self-love and respect for all others and for all forms of life" (Chinn, 1987/1997, p. 135). Chinn's writings in the late 1980s steadfastly maintained her thesis about the insufficiency of merely "gender-sensitive knowledge," asserting that "at this point in history, women's experience must be a central focus in order to begin to reach a point of integrating female and male experience" (Chinn, 1987/1997, pp. 133–134). Further, Chinn conceived of feminist theorizing as an explicitly optimistic project urging that an integral part of emancipatory, social justice struggles in the nursing profession is the preservation of hope among nurses in the face of the technocratic, inhumane health service provision and an articulation of an ideal vision of nursing practice (Chinn, 1997; Kagan et al., 2014, p. 1). Chinn's (1995, 1999; Wheeler & Chinn, 1984) position confronting male dominance and patriarchal oppression of women and aiming for the liberation of women's voices has inspired many followers in the discipline of nursing.

The following passage by Chinn (1999) passionately weaves together a preferred image of nursing:

> Nursing's plans, visions, and dreams for health care appear in many forms. . . . The dreams reflect what is associated with the feminine – yearning for a context or environment that promotes health, healing, and wholeness; recognition of the importance of time spent with another human being nurturing

and encouraging growth and healing; valuing a kind of caring that affirms the uniqueness and individuality of every experience; holding and protecting the person's rights, culture, and values. . . . The reality of what nurses face in practice reflects a system that arises from philosophical viewpoints that have typically eschewed that which is feminine. Nurses are left to dream their dreams, hope for what might be, and ultimately to forsake, even forget, that which could rise to their passion to act.

(p. 464)

This imagery, with its futuristic, hopeful orientation and the centrality of "the feminine" or a uniquely women's experience became a defining thread of nursing feminist discourse in ANS during the period under study. In contrast, few publications problematized the notion of caring in light of class and gender societal dynamics and thus complicated the assumption of women's universal experience (David Allen et al., 1991; McCormick et al., 1998). This minority of writers in the American nursing literature questioned the supposed singularity of "women's voice," suggesting that American nursing theory, claiming to represent "all nursing," obscures the class, gender, and ethnic background of its authors (Thompson, 1992).

Considering Chinn's unequivocal anti-patriarchal feminist stance and a focus on praxis defined as "professional practice directed by and towards social justice goals and outcomes – which include reflexivity, action, and transformation" (Kagan et al., 2014, p. 1) moved by emancipatory aspirations, it is not surprising that ANS became *the* venue for American scholarship based on Jurgen Habermas's critical theory, Paolo Freire's liberation pedagogy, and selected feminist writings. It is in the pages of ANS too that (mostly American) nursing works identified by the authors as postmodern and post-structural have appeared. Up to the end of year 2010, 30 papers in ANS referred to postmodern or post-structural theory, often citing Foucault (Table A1 in the Appendix). The first reference to post-structuralism in ANS was made by Dzurec (1989) when she drew on Foucault's notion of subjugated knowledges to advocate "multiple paradigms for nursing research."

It might appear that the problematic assumption about scientific disciplines having a pyramid structure was avoided in the discourse of nursing science in ANS due to the journal's explicit focus on "practice-oriented models" and an acceptance of theories from other disciplines. But was this so? True, the vision of nursing science in ANS had been open to interdisciplinary influences. Rather than rejecting borrowed ideas, the journal recognized their potential for enriching nursing scholarship. Further, the journal's emancipatory agenda "asserting that all persons, regardless of hierarchy, status, or privilege, should have full access in sharing awareness and participating in social processes" (Kagan et al., 2014, p. 1) had influenced just what kind of borrowed theory was most relevant, namely emancipatory strands of feminism and critical theory of Habermas and Freire. At the same time, ANS's explicit focus on middle-range and practice theory was still grounded in a level-of-abstractness conception of theory. Understandings of what constitutes a concept, a process of concept analysis, metaparadigm as a unifying focus of the discipline, and procedures for deriving middle-range theories, all commonly displayed in ANS publications, echoed the logical positivist and formal-sociological influences. The practice of foregrounding the author's "theoretical framework" and the jargon of models and paradigms continually reinforced what counted as legitimate theoretical discourse in nursing.

A Survey of Postmodern and Post-structural Work in ANS

A survey of postmodern and post-structural articles in ANS through the 1990s and early 2000s reveals a diversity of application of these continental philosophical ideas by mostly American nurse scholars. We find discussions of pedagogical approaches (Ironside, 2001), clinical pathways (Georges & McGuire, 2004), and leadership styles (Reinhardt, 2004). However, references to postmodernism, post-structuralism, or Foucault in these articles as well as in several other (Bent, 1999; Cotton, 2003; Kendall et al., 2003) are quite marginal.

In the following review (based on material in Table A1), I move through numerous examples: papers focused on specific health conditions, writings advocating epistemic diversity in our discipline, and methodological discussions of "postmodern feminism." I aim to show how these applications of postmodern and post-structural ideas in ANS reinforced established concerns of American nursing science (e.g. contesting "traditional" science and medicine in a heavy-handed manner) or contributed to the discourse of "emancipation" within the extended, integrated framework of "nursing's ways of knowing." Notably, these ways of reading Foucault did not challenge established beliefs of American "nursing knowledge" but conformed to them. I then contrast this collection of papers with a few other ANS Foucault-informed publications by the enclave authors: Drevdahl (1999a; 2002), Powers (2003), Cloyes (2006), and Phillips (2001; Phillips & Drevdahl, 2003) whom I position *outside the matrix* based on their critique of some of the key concepts founding American nursing science.

Foucault = Nursing Epistemic Diversity + Emancipation of Women

Two ANS papers with a clinical focus drawing on Foucault's notion of discourse showed how medical, social, and cultural discourses of menopause (Dickson, 1990) and anorexia nervosa (Hardin, 2003a) powerfully shape women's experiences of these conditions. Doering (1992) countered existing power relations between medicine and nursing. Further, echoing Dzurec's (1989) pioneering paper, a recurrent Foucault-inspired theme was contrasting "dominant" versus "marginal discourses" in nursing science – namely, empiricism versus phenomenology (Dzurec, 2003) or Enlightenment science versus postmodernism (Georges, 2003) – and an invitation to embrace "epistemic diversity" (Georges, 2003) or "multiple ways of knowing" (Dzurec, 2003). In different ways, these papers contested the notion of a single truth, namely, the medical model or scientific method whether on the hospital unit or in the nursing classroom and advocated a recognition of the multiplicity of approaches.

These examples (and others discussed in the following) were a marked "improvement" on the kinds of "postmodern" writings examined in the previous chapter. First, Foucault's critique of the clinical gaze made nurses aware of the fragmenting effects of such a gaze and encouraged an exploration into how nursing's approach might be different. Similarly, Foucault's argument that science can be understood as an enhancement of power rather than as a disinterested search for truth heightened nurses' vigilance about the potential effects of "dominant science" on other "ways of knowing" in nursing. Second, these examples drawn from *ANS* undoubtedly find their counterparts in writings by non-American nurses, particularly critiques of medical discourses in relation to (a) how individuals make sense of and experience their illnesses; and (b) how nurses are socialized to think about nursing. And third, among these examples of *ANS* papers we do not find such extravagant deployments (and misrepresentations) of postmodernism and Foucault's ideas as we encountered in the writings of Watson (1995, 1999), Reed (1995), and Polifroni (2010). However, the authors' application of postmodern and post-structural ideas in the majority of *ANS* papers that I examine in this section in some ways continued the practices we encountered in the previous chapter, namely, a shallow reading of postmodern and post-structural literature with the purpose of enhancing epistemological discourses already established in the American nursing science, most notably, a contestation of traditional science and medicine.

Another kind of "postmodern" discussion in *ANS* involved the notion of emancipation articulated with references to feminism (Falk Rafael, 1997; Glass & Davis, 1998; Ogle & Glass, 2006), Habermas (Falk Rafael, 1997), or Freire (Hall, 1999). Although the number of *ANS* papers that refer to both feminism and postmodernism/Foucault is very limited (i.e. I list four papers here, of which three are authored by non-Americans), I go to some length in my discussion of feminism. This is because the discourse of feminism was highly visible in *ANS*. Put another way, I am curious about the disjuncture between the long history of feminist discourse in *ANS* (since at least the early 1980s nurse authors in *ANS*, e.g. MacPherson, 1981, cite feminist literature) and the paucity of postmodern/post-structural feminist writings in this journal. Indeed, it was only in the work of the enclave group nurses where the postmodern variety of feminism was taken up in a robust way.

This is how nurse researchers perceived the emancipatory mechanism of their postmodern feminist approaches: Oral history interviews expose patriarchal power relations and empower nurse participants to transform their realities of public health nursing practice (Falk Rafael, 1997) or female nurses participating in the study speak from their experience and find their voice (Glass & Davis, 1998). The authors explained that postmodern and post-structural literature guided their methodologies in the following ways. First, it helped them to reject positivistic notions of universal truth and to attune to "multiple subjectivities and truths." Second, it gave voice to disadvantaged groups (some authors begin with a "feminist premise" that women are oppressed in patriarchal societies such as ours). Finally, it built an egalitarian researcher–participant relationship and avoided imposing a researcher's interpretation on participants' views.

When these ANS publications advanced a *postmodern feminist* perspective, what they usually meant was *not* a postmodern *wave* of feminist theory or third-wave criticisms of the preceding essentializing varieties of feminist practices. Rather, this perspective amounted to a (second-wave) feminist *add-on* to Foucault's ideas without an attempt to think through serious contradictions between these theoretical positions. In other words, nurse authors proposed emancipatory feminist theory as a supplement to a non-normative and non-agential theorizing of power in Foucault's earlier work. What this "addition" accomplished was the preservation of "the subject" of feminist theory (a woman, a nurse) and her "authentic voice" while recognizing a "multiplicity of women's truths" seen as a sign of postmodernism. Crucially, what this "addition" ignored was the scepticism expressed by postmodern, post-structural, and post-human feminist theorists about the very conception of an authentic female subject.

Alternatively, some nurses more readily accepted Foucault's later work seen as reinstating human agency and its role in social transformation, thus creating a point of synergy with Habermas's theory (e.g. Falk Rafael, 1997). When late, "agential" Foucault was used by nurse authors, a *corrective* was still required for his postmodern "euro- and androcentric perspective. For this reason, feminist theories provide a useful counterbalance" (Falk Rafael, 1997, p. 37). Those ANS discussions (Glass & Davis, 1998; Ogle & Glass, 2006) better informed by interdisciplinary feminist debates, particularly disagreements *within* the feminist movement generated by the postmodern politics of difference, still pivoted around constructing an "integrated" solution able to take into consideration both the anti-oppression, "emancipatory impulse" and postmodern attention to differences.

These works described by the authors as "postmodern feminism" thus cohered with the preferred readings of feminist theory prevalent throughout the journal's history. This established feminist nursing discourse in ANS sought to retrieve that which was unique about women's experiences. Nurse authors did this through unmasking what they presented as inherently masculine scientific ideals of "power, control, instrumentation, . . . logic, objectivity, hard data" said to contradict many values of women-centred science (Chinn, 1985/1996, p. 48); recovering the old gynocentric scientific practices from the male-dominated, patriarchal Western scientific tradition; articulating unique nurses' ways of knowing in the health care system colonized by technology and biomedicine; and reclaiming feminist, "femicentric" approaches to nursing research from "critical social theory"–guided approaches "developed by men in a period of history when androcentrism dominated academic thought" (J. Campbell & Bunting, 1991/1999, p. 411).

A concurrent line of thought in some nursing feminist writings in ANS was an emphasis on the desirability of "idealism" and optimism understood as promoting "hope for a better future for women and for all" (J. Campbell & Bunting,

1991/1999, p. 416). Such nursing feminist writings typical of *ANS* focused on sharpening, strategically or unwittingly, the binaries of androcentric/gynocentric and masculine/feminine. In contrast, arguments in wider feminist literature reprinted in nursing textbooks (e.g. Fox Keller, 1978/1999) about a highly problematic tendency to ascribe an inherent masculinity to science (and medicine) did not appear to trouble the discourse of feminism in *ANS* during those years. In addition, some nurses' focus on a separatist version of feminism obscured any serious attention to the world of interdisciplinary feminist theory with its multiplying directions.

Cursorily, Chinn (1995) acknowledged a presence in nursing literature of a variety of feminist influences: liberal feminism concerned with legal rights for women, "critical social feminism" problematizing the assumptions of women's universal experience based on recognition of class and ethnicity categories alongside the category of gender, ecofeminism establishing a parallel between patriarchal exploitation of women and nature, and post-structural feminism described by Chinn as concerned with deconstructing gender dichotomies presented in language. Despite this variety, Chinn identified "cultural feminism" focused on the experiences of women and aiming at women's liberation from patriarchal and oppressive forces as most closely aligned with nursing's goals.

Clearly, these various directions in American nursing feminist discourse developed under an interdisciplinary influence. Sandra Harding (1986/1999), a scientist and feminist critic of science often cited in nursing literature, writing in the mid-1980s, usefully summarized two key directions in broad American feminist literature that emerged as alternatives to strongly criticized Western science: postmodern feminism (e.g. drawing on nonfeminist critics of the Enlightenment science such as Nietzsche, Derrida, Foucault, Lacan, Rorty, and Gadamer) and the feminist standpoint. Harding (1986/1999) writes,

> At its best postmodernism envisions epistemology in a world where thought does not need policing. It recognizes the existence today of far less than the ideal speech situation, but disregards (or fails to acknowledge) the political struggles necessary to bring about change.[4] The standpoint tendency attempts to move us toward that ideal world by legitimating and empowering the "subjugated knowledges" of women. . . . [But] It fails nonetheless to challenge the modernist intimacies between knowledge and power, or the legitimacy of assuming there can be a single, feminist story of reality.
>
> (p. 403)

Continental philosophers whom Harding calls "nonfeminist postmodernists" have pointed out a constitutive link between power and knowledge as well as the problematic nature of metanarratives claiming to speak on behalf of all. These central insights complicate some feminist imaginings of the world characterized by a democratic ideal of (women's) communicative rationality where all women can exercise their unrestrained "voice" and speak from a unified perspective. Harding argues that feminism will benefit from keeping these contradictory tendencies in play and refusing to choose either of them. In other words, in contrast to feminist projects that seek to stabilize the analytical categories of feminist theory, she perceives their instability as a necessary condition for theoretical projects, if they are to be of any practical significance, to be able to account for the social experiences of women in the contemporary world.

When the qualifier *postmodern* was added to *feminism* in ANS, it was still the futuristic-optimistic and "uniquely women's" strand of feminism that emerged in these writings. Foucault was simply added as a coat of paint on a fixed picture of (second-wave) feminist nursing ideas. His ideas did not destabilize any of the categories of nursing feminism in the way Harding, in the previous quotation, described they did in wider feminist theory. As well, no attempt was made by nurse authors to keep the contradictory lines of feminist thought in play, but rather the opposite tendency was in evidence – to integrate them, to devise a *coherent* framework where the emancipatory telos dominated.

I suggest that the legitimacy of a "postmodern feminist" theoretical discourse in ANS often seemed to depend on a compulsory welding of (conflicting) theoretical positions of anti-patriarchal feminism (a line of thought well established in ANS, e.g. David, 2000) and of postmodernism. That postmodernism would be equally incredulous of the metanarratives of "traditional" science *and* of the notion of patriarchal domination presupposing a generic identity of an (oppressed) female nurse, female patient, and female nurse theorist was not the kind of insight generated in postmodern feminist writings in ANS. In other words, feminist theory in ANS was mostly represented by second-wave feminism, although it was rarely acknowledged as such. Explicit criticisms of this theoretical position by later generations of feminists (e.g. postmodern and post-humanist feminists) were a rare occurrence in this journal. It appears that not only ANS, but American nursing literature at large circulated second-wave, emancipatory feminist ideas while postmodern feminism was rarely acknowledged in a meaningful way (for an exception see Rodgers, 2005, p. 167; Sandelowski writing on technology [2002; Barnard & Sandelowski, 2001]; and the enclave scholars Drevdahl, 1999a, 1999b; Phillips, 2001; Thompson, 1992).

Thus, the majority of ANS papers claiming postmodern and post-structural orientation hardly departed from the well-established concerns in American nursing metatheory to establish nursing science as separate and different from Western science and medicine. What distinguished postmodern and post-structural writings in ANS from those discussed in the previous chapter is that in ANS, a number of articles linked Foucault's ideas to a version of feminism positing the subject of a female nurse engaged in emancipatory praxis against the oppressive patriarchal medical model and in a benevolent empowerment of her patients.

Outside the Matrix: Interrogating the Notions of the Person, Empowerment, and Experience

In contrast to articles in ANS claiming postmodern and post-structural orientation and reviewed thus far, we find a few analyses distinguished by a perceptive reading of postmodern and post-structural theory and dealing with a set of questions starkly removed from the previously identified concerns. I describe this reading of post-structural work as open-ended in the sense that it did not seek to conform to established discourses of nursing knowledge but rather, in a spirit of scholarship *and* in a spirit of radical French influences, sought to reread the (Western, white, middle-class) nursing theoretical canon. Rather than aiming to fortify the theoretical discourses of nursing science and of feminist methodologies as they were conceived in other ANS publications, these analyses turned their critical attention precisely to those established ways of thinking.

Drawing on postmodern feminist criticisms of the unitary self, essentialism, agency, and subjectivity, Denise Drevdahl (1999a) challenged nursing's conceptualization of the person. She put on trial not only the grand narrative of Western medicine but equally the grand narrative of "the whole generic person" of nursing theory. "The unitary human being, in the end, only comes about through the suppression and denial of differences," Drevdahl (1999a, p. 4) asserted. Much nursing theory, she explained, has been written from the position of a white, middle-class person, and thus its appeal to the whole generic person disregards interactions among the individual's race, class, and sex. "Nursing ideas and theories do not, and cannot, exist outside of class, race, political, and other social processes. Yet, these processes curiously are absent from the discipline's conceptual frameworks" (p. 5), wrote Drevdahl. Further, an egalitarian conception of the nurse–patient relationship does not recognize a constitutive role of power. Individualistic assumptions of nursing theory mask systematic, institutionalized oppression. "Nursing theorists have offered little information about how the social or cultural is constituted, how it is to be understood, or how the social or cultural information collected about the person is to be [interpreted]" (p. 4). Thus, Drevdahl did not attempt to assimilate postmodern feminist ideas to the existing understandings of the person as a nursing metaparadigm concept, but rather she undermined the foundational assumptions about this concept operative in nursing theories.

Drevdahl and others went beyond pointing out the limitations of nursing's theoretical conceptions. Applying Derrida's notion of binaries and Foucault's conception of power/knowledge, they analysed "the complexities of language in relation to race" and advanced an anti-essentialist understanding of gender and race as constitutive elements of nursing practice (Phillips & Drevdahl, 2003, p. 17). In another paper, Drevdahl (2002) problematized a romantic vision of "community" common in nursing literature. She invited readers "to see the contradictions of community – that is, community being both home (a location of refuge, similitude, and familiarity) and border (a place of peril, difference, and unfamiliarity)" (pp. 9–10).

Penny Powers, another American author, problematized the notion of *patient empowerment* held in high regard in nursing literature and posited as an ideal for nursing practice (despite disagreements about how empowerment is achieved due to conflicting conceptualizations of power itself). Powers observed that empowerment is overwhelmingly assumed to be successful when the patient's actions align with nurses' goals. But, Powers asked, how is this different from coercion? Of course, a nurse acts without direct force, in line with her professional codes of ethics, but her professional responsibility nevertheless compels her to "empower" the patient towards a *certain* end. Powers relied on Foucault's ideas to tease out what empowerment entails. The nurse is involved in the practice of governmentality, explained by Foucault as governing the conduct of others (Powers, 2003).

Methodological papers by Debby Phillips (2001) and Kristin Cloyes (2006) were informed by Foucault's theorizing of power/knowledge and Judith Butler's work on gender. Phillips (2001) studied discursive constructions of masculinity to understand and challenge male violence. Refreshingly, the author viewed this phenomenon as social, and as such, mediated through language. (Male) subjectivities are understood as discursively, culturally produced and a result of performativity. Phillips analysed media narratives and interview data using current methods of social psychology sensitive to feminist postmodern theorizing of subjectivities. Significantly, the author implicitly challenged naturalistic notions of maleness and femaleness prevalent in feminist writings in ANS and invited nurses to understand nursing practices as socially embedded.

Cloyes (2006) described her approach to analysing interview texts generated during her ethnographic study on a prison unit for offenders with severe mental illness. She treated

> interview data as texts that are, like other genres of discursive production, rhetorically powerful acts . . . where people signify, negotiate, and perform identity and agency in a local, highly specific context: a prison control unit that is characterized by an intersection of psychiatric and prison discourse.
> (p. 89)

Cloyes drew attention to the socially grounded textual production of both interview texts and research reports, and thus foregrounded issues of discourse, representation, and interpretation involved in any (social) practice of research. This stance, Cloyes claimed, allowed her to avoid two issues. One was the simplistic adherence to the words of participants, whereby the "critical paradigm" of nursing research involving marginalized groups "sanctifies" the "voice" and "experience" of research participants as a mechanism to ensure research ethics. The other was the opposite – further marginalization of research participants. Cloyes enlisted Foucault's notion of the care of the self as an ethical position of the researcher – "the relation one has to (and with) oneself" (p. 88) – as enabling her to "present an account of prisoners diagnosed with mental illness [in such a way] that emphasizes their agency and participation in control unit discourse" (p. 95).

Published in ANS and intelligently informed by postmodern and post-structural ideas, these few papers (Cloyes, 2006; Drevdahl, 1999a; Phillips, 2001; Powers, 2003) can be contrasted with other applications of French theory in ANS. In these papers, the practice of theorizing adheres neither to a discourse of unique nursing science nor to a discourse of emancipatory praxis founded upon the naturalized image of a nurse. (Yet moral and ethical concerns of these postmodern writings are evident, addressing an ever-present quibble about the incompatibility of Foucault and nursing.) More than that, the articles challenge these two cornerstones of the theoretical discourse in *ANS*. Rhetorically, by not exploiting the tropes of models, levels of theory, and (meta)paradigms to legitimate their place within the "disciplinary structure of nursing knowledge," the authors demonstrate an alternative practice of theorizing in the discipline of nursing in the United States. Substantively, by interrogating the foundational assumptions of nursing theory and the language of "experience" in nursing research (e.g. the nature of the person, the nature of nursing represented in American nursing theory as an ahistorical, non-social entity transcending the realities of gender, race, class, and power in nurse–patient relations) the authors engaged in the politics of disciplinary knowledge production. In other words, they exposed "nursing foundations" as rooted in specific assumptions and thus as contestable; in a post-structuralist vein they attempted to de-naturalize the category of "foundational disciplinary knowledge."

As the foregoing discussion suggests, the use of postmodern and post-structural ideas in the U.S. leading theoretical nursing journal *ANS* demonstrated a marked diversity of topics, genres (e.g. argument, methodological discussion), and the effects of drawing on Foucault's work. Beyond any doubt, in the first decade of the 21st century, *ANS* was a leading nursing voice for critical scholarship including post-structural writings in the United States. Notably, in January 2003, a thematic issue of *ANS* was devoted to "Critical and Postmodern Perspectives." Several publications cited throughout this chapter (i.e. Dzurec, 2003; Georges, 2003; Hardin, 2003a; Phillips & Drevdahl, 2003) appeared in that issue. Attention to interdisciplinary French theory in an American nursing science journal was a reason for enthusiasm, even if it was short-lived. In *ANS*, references to postmodernism, post-structuralism, or Foucault effectively disappeared after 2010.[5]

The Enclave Group

Interestingly, American nurse scholars whose work I have singled out as providing insightful readings of postmodern and post-structural theory (i.e. Cloyes, Drevdahl, Hardin, Phillips, Powers) were all connected to the Nursing Program at the University of Washington. Some of these authors in their publications acknowledged the supervisory role of David Allen. As early as the mid-1980s, Allen began introducing into nursing theoretical literature Habermas's work, hermeneutics, and feminist theory. Throughout the 1990s, he appeared to be instrumental in establishing and co-convening the annual International Critical and Feminist Perspectives in Nursing conference.

Another nurse scholar, Janice Thompson, then a professor of nursing at the University of Southern Maine, has played an important role in spearheading this conference and contributing to the discussions informed by postmodern feminist thought in relation to the politics of difference. To help the reader appreciate the avant-garde thinking of this scholar, I will summarize her earlier paper in *ANS* (Thompson, 1985).

Thompson (1985) invited nurses to advance nursing science beyond both the empiricism of Hempel much criticized by nurses *and* the historicism of Kuhn and Laudan well respected by nurses. She identified both of these philosophy of science perspectives as comprising "a distinctly American view of the situation in contemporary philosophy" (p. 60), suggesting that *continental* philosophy carried an unexplored potential for nursing scholarship. Thompson introduced the antifoundationalist ideas of Habermas and Hans-Georg Gadamer that undermined the dominant view of a legitimate science espoused in nursing literature. Drawing on these philosophical works, Thompson urged nurses to expand their horizons of scholarship. The most striking move, which set Thompson's critique apart from common assaults on "empiricism" to elevate "nursing theory" and even more informed views that recognized the benefits of the historicist tradition in science, was her use of the antifoundationalist continental ideas to *critique* nursing theory. Although Thompson's critique was partly directed against the "scientific method of the nurse scientist program" (an approach advocated by nurse scientists like Gortner), it was equally aimed at nurse theorists' attempts to define foundations of nursing, for example, through concept analysis. Prefiguring some aspects of Risjord's (2010) critique, Thompson's paper recognized nursing "conceptual schemes" like Roy's, Orem's, Rogers's, and Parse's as part of the logical empiricist legacy and rebuked the pyramid image of foundationalist science (p. 62). Refreshingly, Thompson did not thrash science but sought to highlight the practical dimension of rationality in science (p. 64).

During the same year, in the nursing journal *Image*, David Allen (1985) similarly drew on Gadamerian hermeneutics and Habermasian types of rationality to introduce "alternative models of science that emphasize understanding and emancipation" (p. 58). Tracing Allen's publications from the 1980s to the early 2000s, we can witness his articulate attempts to intervene in American nursing theory. Strategically deploying the tropes of "nursing science," he introduced ideas capable of undermining the very theoretical project such conceived. Allen engaged in a kind of dance or balancing act in attempting to be heard in "nursing science/nursing theory" circles while trying to challenge their understanding of science and theory. Nurse scholars Cloyes, Drevdahl, Hardin, Phillips, and Powers were all connected to the University of Washington and appear to have been mentored (as I can judge from the acknowledgements in the articles) by David Allen and/or Janice Thompson.

In the early 2000s, these authors actively pursued publication opportunities in non-U.S. nursing journals – *Nursing Inquiry*, *Nursing Philosophy*, and *Journal of Advanced Nursing* (Allen, 2006; Allen & Cloyes, 2005; Allen & Hardin, 2001; Cloyes, 2007; Hardin, 2001, 2003b, 2003c; Phillips, 2005). These papers continued post-structural critiques of "whiteness" in nursing and of the notion of meaning and the language of experience widely accepted in nursing literature. The majority of publications by these scholars fell between the years 2001 and 2007, mostly in *Nursing Inquiry*.

Criticisms of subjectivity, language, and power based on perceptive readings of postmodern and post-structural theory in the small set of *ANS* papers that

I described as located "outside the American nursing theory matrix" likely have had *no* effect on a wider understanding of French theory in American nursing scholarship and, even more importantly, *no* effect on the conception of nursing theory in the American discourse of unique nursing science. On the other hand, a plethora of American nursing theory textbooks exerted a wide-reaching effect on "nursing knowledge" in the United States by reproducing problematic use and interpretations of postmodern and post-structural theory. Table A2 summarizes references to postmodernism and post-structuralism in multi-edition nursing theory textbooks by Chinn and Kramer (2004, 2011), Johnson and Webber (2010), Meleis (1997, 2007, 2012), and L. O. Walker and Avant (2011) among others.

Concluding Thoughts

Continental philosophical ideas and writings, selectively taken up by American nurse scholars, have produced peculiar intersections with nursing metatheoretical and "nursing theory" discourses. The most surprising observation that triggered my study was a relative invisibility of postmodern and post-structural ideas in the U.S. nursing literature as compared to French theory's much wider reception and acceptance in other English-language nursing publications (e.g. Table A3 lists non-American books citing Foucault). American nurse authors seemed to engage with postmodern and post-structural theory less than their non-American counterparts did and also seemed to engage differently (as the next chapter further demonstrates).

In this chapter, I continued to survey the intersections between influential nursing metatheoretical perspectives and broadly postmodern ideas. The question answered in this chapter was, How have postmodern and post-structural sensibilities, tangible across academic fields in the last decades of the 20th century, played out in American nursing scholarship, particularly in the leading theoretical journal, *ANS*?

Locked in the discourse of nursing science (and moreover, the unacknowledged and unrecognized view of science trapped in logical positivism), the viability of postmodern and post-structural ideas in the American nursing theory literature has been severely limited. It is ironic that when American nurse academics gathered for the first theory conference in 1967, it was only a year after French theory entered the United States and started its consequential journey from the Johns Hopkins University humanities conference. Hidden in literature departments, French theory did not have much chance to intersect with nurse scientists in the 1960s–1980s. But even when a discourse of nursing theory overlapped with the discourses of nursing research and philosophy (e.g. as reflected in the pluralistic, integrative conception of nursing science in *ANS*), these intersections between nursing theory and interdisciplinary theory were strictly codified by nursing writing conventions and the prevailing rhetoric of "nursing science" and "theoretical frameworks." A strong and lasting focus on ideas of oppression and emancipation screened out theoretical perspectives sceptical of such intentions (or, at least, presenting a more complex picture of power and subjugation). The most interesting and rigorous nursing postmodern and post-structural works illustrated in this chapter by the enclave group questioned the foundational assumptions of nursing theory but were seemingly powerless to disturb the status quo in the best-known "nursing knowledge" texts.[6]

Notes

1 Not only does the intellectual matrix passively exclude certain philosophical ideas, making them marginal and invisible, it also actively produces unintelligibility via an "additive," cumulative mode of inclusion. Only that which is both included into the matrix and made alike with its other elements is legitimated and gains intelligibility. It seems that as long as the American nursing theory matrix (i.e. the structure of nursing knowledge à la Fawcett, the patterns of knowing à la Chinn, the models of theory development à la L. O. Walker and Avant) dominates the discipline's theoretical imagination, contemporary continental philosophy/social theory will remain in a lose–lose situation in American theoretical discourse.

2 Jonas-Simpson (2004), a humanbecoming scholar, in her review in NSQ identified Chinn and Kramer's conception of nursing science grounded in "ways of knowing" (rather than in existing nursing conceptual frameworks such as the humanbecoming theory) as a limitation of this otherwise commendable text. For an alternative criticism of Chinn and Kramer's depiction of nursing knowledge, particularly their separation of "empirics" from "ethics" and a proposal of empirical ways to evaluate "personal" and "ethical" knowing, see Risjord (2011, pp. 500–501).

3 Although these editorial trends in the journal may continue, I use the past tense here and elsewhere in the chapter because my study focuses mostly on a period ending in 2010, and I do not want to make assumptions about the journal after that date.

4 This statement can be contested by pointing out actual political engagement of several French theorists. However, Harding expresses a prevailing sentiment that indeed represents postmodernism as politically uncommitted.

5 A CINAHL search in March 2022 using variations of keywords *postmodernism, poststructuralism,* or *Foucault* in All Text, for articles published in *Advances in Nursing Science* from January 2011 to the end of 2021 produced a meagre four hits: three by Canadian authors and one by an American author, all from 2018 to 2020.

6 A textbook on "emancipatory nursing," edited by American authors Kagan et al. (2014), provides a peculiar common ground for several nursing perspectives: for some scholars of the enclave group (Drevdahl, Phillips), Canadian and Australian Foucauldian scholars (Perron, Rudge, Gagnon), and American nurse theorists and metatheoreticians (M. C. Smith, Watson, Chinn, Meleis). This commonality, however, is founded upon specific exclusions dictated by the goal of "emancipation" and discussed in this chapter: Post-structural ideas are assimilated as long as their point of application is the topic of male violence against women or the nurses' ethical self-work enabling them to speak truth to power. Overall, however, this anthology is a step in a right direction. It is a better way of presenting post-structural and Foucault-informed nursing scholarship than through synthetic projects such as those by Roy and Jones (2007) or Chinn and Kramer (2011, 2015).

References

Allen, D. G. (1985). Nursing research and social control: Alternate models of science that emphasize understanding and emancipation. *Image: The Journal of Nursing Scholarship,* 17(2), 58–64.

Allen, D. G. (2006). Whiteness and difference in nursing. *Nursing Philosophy, 7*(2), 65–78.

Allen, D. G., Allman, K. K., & Powers, P. (1991). Feminist nursing research without gender. *Advances in Nursing Science, 13*(3), 49–58.

Allen, D. G., & Cloyes, K. (2005). The language of "experience" in nursing research. *Nursing Inquiry, 12*(2), 98–105.

Allen, D. G., & Hardin, P. (2001). Discourse analysis and the epidemiology of meaning. *Nursing Philosophy, 2*(2), 163–176.

Ashley, J. A. (1976). *Hospitals, paternalism, and the role of the nurse.* Teachers College Press, Columbia University.

Barnard, A., & Sandelowski, M. (2001). Technology and humane nursing care: (Ir)reconcilable or invented difference. *Journal of Advanced Nursing, 34*(3), 367–375.

Benner, P. (1985). Quality of life: A phenomenological perspective on explanation, prediction, and understanding of nursing science. *Advances in Nursing Science, 8*, 1–14.

Bent, K. (1999). Seeking the both/and of a nursing research proposal. *Advances in Nursing Science, 21*(3), 76–89.

Campbell, J. C., & Bunting, S. (1999). Voices and paradigms: Perspectives on critical and feminist theory in nursing. In E. C. Polifroni & M. Welch (Eds.), *Perspectives on philosophy of science in nursing: An historical and contemporary anthology* (pp. 411–422). Lippincott Williams & Wilkins. (Original work published in *Advances in Nursing Science, 13*(3), 1–15, in 1991)

Carper, B. (1978). Fundamental patterns of knowing in nursing. *Advances in Nursing Science, 1*(1), 13–23.

Chinn, P. L. (1995). Feminism and nursing. *Annual Review of Nursing Research, 13*(1), 267–289.

Chinn, P. L. (1996). Debunking myths in nursing theory and research. In J. W. Kenney (Ed.), *Philosophical and theoretical perspectives for advanced nursing practice* (pp. 47–55). Jones and Bartlett Publishers. (Original work published in *Image: Journal of Nursing Scholarship, 17*(2), 45–49, in 1985)

Chinn, P. L. (1997a). Response: ReVision and passion. In L. H. Nicoll (Ed.), *Perspectives on nursing theory* (3rd ed., pp. 133–136). Lippincott. (Original work published in *Scholarly Inquiry for Nursing Practice, 1*(1), 21–24, in 1987)

Chinn, P. L. (1997b). Response to "Ethics and the geography of the nurse–patient relationship." *Scholarly Inquiry for Nursing Practice, 11*(1), 61–63.

Chinn, P. L. (1999). Gender and nursing science. In E. C. Polifroni & M. Welch (Eds.), *Perspectives on philosophy of science in nursing* (pp. 462–466). Lippincott.

Chinn, P. L. (n.d.). "Projects" tab, "Cassandra." https://peggychinn.com/projects/cassandra/

Chinn, P. L., & Jacobs, M. K. (1978). A model for theory development in nursing. *Advances in Nursing Science, 1*(1), 1–11.

Chinn, P. L., & Kramer, M. K. (2004). *Integrated knowledge development in nursing* (6th ed.). Mosby.

Chinn, P. L., & Kramer, M. K. (2008). *Integrated theory and knowledge development in nursing* (7th ed.). Mosby Elsevier.

Chinn, P. L., & Kramer, M. K. (2011). *Integrated theory and knowledge development in nursing* (8th ed.). Elsevier Mosby.

Chinn, P. L., & Kramer, M. K. (2015). *Knowledge development in nursing: Theory and process* (9th ed.). Elsevier Health Sciences.

Cloyes, K. G. (2006). An ethic of analysis: An argument for critical analysis of research interviews as an ethical practice. *Advances in Nursing Science, 29*(2), 84–97.

Cloyes, K. G. (2007). Prisoners signify: A political discourse analysis of mental illness in a prison control unit. *Nursing Inquiry, 14*(3), 202–211.

Cotton, A. (2003). The discursive field of web-based health research: Implications for nursing research in cyberspace. *Advances in Nursing Science, 26*(4), 307–319.

David, B. A. (2000). Nursing's gender politics: Reformulating the footnotes. *Advances in Nursing Science, 23*(1), 83–93.

Dickson, G. L. (1990). A feminist poststructuralist analysis of the knowledge of menopause. *Advances in Nursing Science, 12*(3), 15–31.

Doering, L. (1992). Power and knowledge in nursing: A feminist poststructuralist view. *Advances in Nursing Science, 14*(4), 24–33.

Drevdahl, D. (1999a). Sailing beyond: Nursing theory and the person. *Advances in Nursing Science, 21*(4), 1–13.

Drevdahl, D. (1999b). Meanings of community in a community health center. *Public Health Nursing, 16*(6), 417–425.

Drevdahl, D. (2002). Home and border: The contradictions of community. *Advances in Nursing Science, 24*(3), 8–20.

Duffy, J. R., & Hoskins, L. M. (2003). The quality-caring model: Blending dual paradigms. *Advances in Nursing Science, 26*(1), 77–88.

Dzurec, L. (1989). The necessity for and evolution of multiple paradigms for nursing research: A poststructuralist perspective. *Advances in Nursing Science, 11*(4), 69–77.

Dzurec, L. (2003). Poststructuralist musings on the mind/body question in health care. *Advances in Nursing Science, 26*(1), 63–76.

Falk Rafael, A. R. (1997). Advocacy oral history: A research methodology for social activism in nursing. *Advances in Nursing Science, 20*(2), 32–44.

Fawcett, J. (1997). The relationship between theory and research: A double helix. In L. H. Nicoll (Ed.), *Perspectives on nursing theory* (3rd ed., pp. 716–725). Lippincott. (Original work published in *Advances in Nursing Science, 1*(1), 49–62, in 1978)

Fox Keller, E. (1999). Gender and science. In E. C. Polifroni & M. Welch (Eds.), *Perspectives on philosophy of science in nursing: An historical and contemporary anthology* (pp. 427–439). Lippincott Williams & Wilkins. (Original work published 1978)

Georges, J. (2003). An emerging discourse: Toward epistemic diversity in nursing. *Advances in Nursing Science, 26*(1), 44–52.

Georges, J., & McGuire, S. (2004). Deconstructing clinical pathways: Mapping the landscape of health care. *Advances in Nursing Science, 27*(1), 2–11.

Glass, N., & Davis, K. (1998). An emancipatory impulse: A feminist postmodern integrated turning point in nursing research. *Advances in Nursing Science, 21*(1), 43–52.

Glass, N., & Davis, K. (2004). Reconceptualizing vulnerability: Deconstruction and reconstruction as a postmodern feminist analytical research method. *Advances in Nursing Science, 27*(2), 82–92.

Hall, J. (1999). Marginalization revisited: Critical, postmodern, and liberation perspectives. *Advances in Nursing Science, 22*(2), 88–102.

Hardin, P. K. (2001). Theory and language: Locating agency between free will and discursive marionettes. *Nursing Inquiry, 8*(1), 11–18.

Hardin, P. K. (2003a). Social and cultural considerations in recovery from anorexia nervosa: A critical poststructuralist analysis. *Advances in Nursing Science, 26*(1), 5–16.

Hardin, P. K. (2003b). Constructing experience in individual interviews, autobiographies and on-line accounts: A poststructuralist approach. *Journal of Advanced Nursing, 41*(6), 536–544.

Hardin, P. K. (2003c). Shape-shifting discourses of anorexia nervosa: Reconstituting psychopathology. *Nursing Inquiry, 10*(4), 209–217.

Harding, S. (1999). The instability of the analytical categories of feminist theory. In E. C. Polifroni & M. Welch (Eds.), *Perspectives on philosophy of science in nursing: An historical and contemporary anthology* (pp. 396–410). Lippincott Williams & Wilkins. (Original work published in *Signs*, 11(4), 645–664, in 1986)

Ironside, P. (2001). Creating a research base for nursing education: An interpretive review of conventional, critical, feminist, postmodern, and phenomenologic pedagogies. *Advances in Nursing Science*, 23(3), 72–87.

Jacobs-Kramer, M. K., & Chinn, P. L. (1997). Perspectives on knowing: A model of nursing knowledge. In L. H. Nicoll (Ed.), *Perspectives on nursing theory* (3rd ed., pp. 323–330). Lippincott. (Original work published in *Scholarly Inquiry for Nursing Practice*, 2, 129–139, in 1988)

Johnson, B. M., & Webber, P. B. (2010). *An introduction to theory and reasoning in nursing* (3rd ed.). Lippincott Williams & Wilkins.

Johnson, J. L. (1991). Nursing science: Basic, applied or practical? Implications for the art of nursing. *Advances in Nursing Science*, 14(1), 7–16.

Jonas-Simpson, C. (2004). Reflections on a new edition of a seminal nursing text. *Nursing Science Quarterly*, 17(4), 356–363.

Kagan, P. N., & Chinn, P. L. (2010). We're all here for the good of the patient: A dialogue on power. *Nursing Science Quarterly*, 23(1), 41–46.

Kagan, P. N., Smith, M. C., & Chinn, P. L. (Eds.). (2014). *Philosophies and practices of emancipatory nursing: Social justice as praxis*. Routledge.

Kendall, J., Hatton, D., Beckett, A., & Leo, M. (2003). Children's accounts of attention-deficit/hyperactivity disorder. *Advances in Nursing Science*, 26(2), 114–130.

MacPherson, K. I. (1981). Menopause as disease: The social construction of a metaphor. *Advances in Nursing Science*, 3(2), 95–113.

McCormick, J., Kirkham, S., & Hayes, V. (1998). Abstracting women: Essentialism in women's health research. *Health Care for Women International*, 19(6), 495–504.

Meleis, A. I. (1997). *Theoretical nursing: Development and progress* (3rd ed.). Lippincott.

Meleis, A. I. (2007). *Theoretical nursing: Development and progress* (4th ed.). Lippincott Williams & Wilkins.

Meleis, A. I. (2012). *Theoretical nursing: Development and progress* (5th ed.). Wolters Kluwer/Lippincott Williams & Wilkins.

Ogle, K. R., & Glass, N. (2006). Mobile subjectivities: Positioning the nonunitary self in critical feminist and postmodern research. *Advances in Nursing Science*, 29(2), 170–180.

Phillips, D. (2001). Methodology for social accountability: Multiple methods and feminist, poststructural, psychoanalytic discourse analysis. *Advances in Nursing Science*, 23(4), 49–66.

Phillips, D. (2005). Reproducing normative and marginalized masculinities: Adolescent male popularity and the outcast. *Nursing Inquiry*, 12(3), 219–230.

Phillips, D., & Drevdahl, D. (2003). "Race" and the difficulties of language. *Advances in Nursing Science*, 26(1), 17–29.

Polifroni, E. C. (2010). Power, right, and truth: Foucault's triangle as a model for clinical power. *Nursing Science Quarterly*, 23(1), 8–12.

Powers, P. (2003). Empowerment as treatment and the role of health professionals. *Advances in Nursing Science*, 26(3), 227–237.

Reed, P. (1995). A treatise on nursing knowledge development for the 21st century: Beyond postmodernism. *Advances in Nursing Science*, 17(3), 70–84.

Reinhardt, A. (2004). Discourse on the transformational leader metanarrative or finding the right person for the job. *Advances in Nursing Science*, 27(1), 21–31.

Risjord, M. (2010). *Nursing knowledge: Science, practice, and philosophy.* Wiley-Blackwell.

Risjord, M. (2011). Nursing science. In F. Gifford (Ed.), *Philosophy of medicine* (pp. 489–522). Elsevier.

Rodgers, B. L. (2005). *Developing nursing knowledge: Philosophical traditions and influences.* Lippincott Williams & Wilkins.

Roy, C., Sr., & Jones, D. A. (Eds.). (2007). *Nursing knowledge development and clinical practice.* Springer Publishing Company.

Sandelowski, M. (2002). Visible humans, vanishing bodies, and virtual nursing: Complications of life, presence, place, and identity. *Advances in Nursing Science, 24*(3), 58–70.

Thompson, J. L. (1985). Practical discourse in nursing: Going beyond empiricism and historicism. *Advances in Nursing Science, 7*(4), 59–71.

Thompson, J. L. (1992). Identity politics, essentialism, and constructions of "home" in nursing. In J. L. Thompson, D. G. Allen, & L. Rodriguez-Fisher (Eds.), *Critique, resistance, and action: Working papers in the politics of nursing* (pp. 21–34). NLN.

Walker, L. O., & Avant, K. C. (2011). *Strategies for theory construction in nursing* (5th ed.). Pearson Prentice Hall.

Watson, J. (1995). Postmodernism and knowledge development in nursing. *Nursing Science Quarterly, 8*(2), 60–64.

Watson, J. (1999). *Postmodern nursing and beyond.* Churchill Livingstone.

Wheeler, C. E., & Chinn, P. L. (1984). *Peace & power: A handbook of feminist process* (1st ed.). Margaretdaughters, Inc.

White, J. (1995). Patterns of knowing: Review, critique, and update. *Advances in Nursing Science, 17*(4), 73–86.

6 Postmodern and Post-structural Ideas in Non-American Nursing Literature

Examining Nurse–Patient Relationships and the Holistic Nurse

In this chapter I present examples of Foucault-informed non-American nursing scholarship. I chose these examples because of their significant difference from the American nursing theory citing postmodern and post-structural writings in the 1990s and 2000s. Indeed, my aim is to sharpen the contrast between the writings generated inside and outside of the matrix of American nursing theory.

As I suggested in Chapters 4 and 5, the contextualization of postmodern and post-structural theory in the philosophy of "unique science" common in American nursing theory obscures the perspective of continental philosophy, from which Foucault and other postmodern and post-structural theorists can be read to a different effect. In this chapter I showcase selected examples of a different kind of nursing scholarship informed by postmodern and post-structural theory where authors view these intellectual movements, implicitly or explicitly, in the context of *continental philosophical* influences upon the humanities and social sciences. What all these examples have in common is that they serve to highlight what is missing in American nursing theory. In other words, they unwittingly "fill," and thus make visible, significant lacunae in American nursing theory claiming postmodern and post-structural influences. They exemplify the intellectual content never thought worthy of attention by American nurse theorists or unable to gain intelligibility within the American nursing's disciplinary matrix. This "unintelligible content" includes Foucault-informed analyses of *nursing practice* and postmodern/post-structural critiques of holistic nursing theory. In other words, whether we agree or disagree with specific arguments and points of view presented by (mostly non-American) writers in these applications of postmodern and post-structural ideas (and my allegiances are made clear through my exposition of these writings), American nursing theory citing postmodernism, post-structuralism, and Foucault has not produced anything comparable to these perceptive applications.[1]

Two such applications are central to this chapter: theorizing of the nurse–patient relationship (May, 1990, 1992a, 1992b, 1995a, 1995b) and an examination of the holistic nurse through a historical lens (Nelson, 2000). Summarizing these high-quality exemplars of postmodern and post-structural work, I draw attention to how May and Nelson embed Foucault's ideas in the context of selected sociological traditions or of historical research – those specific academic

DOI: 10.4324/9781003194439-6

domains already broadly informed by continental philosophical concerns – rather than in the context of Western philosophy of science *and* American philosophy of nursing science. The cases discussed in this chapter opened new vistas for understanding nursing practice and nursing knowledge as socially and historically contingent phenomena.

But before presenting these cases, I provide an overview of this substantial area of nursing literature during roughly the first two decades of its existence. The first references to Foucault occurred almost simultaneously in the late 1980s in the British journal, *Journal of Advanced Nursing* (*JAN*; Lees et al., 1987; Chapman, 1988) and in the American journal *Advances in Nursing Science* (*ANS*; Dzurec, 1989). Over the ensuing 20–25 years, hundreds of articles and numerous book chapters, anthologies, and monographs in English cited Foucault and other philosophers working in postmodern and post-structural traditions. The overwhelming majority of these publications were authored by nurses outside of the United States and appeared in three journals: *JAN*, *Nursing Inquiry* (*NI*; established in 1994 under Australian editorship and with a noticeable Foucauldian orientation), and *Nursing Philosophy* (*NP*; established in the year 2000). Table A3 in the Appendix provides information and summaries of selected textbooks and book chapters by non-American nurses and social scientists writing in nursing.

During this period, non-American Anglophone nursing scholarship informed by postmodern and post-structural theory was voluminous and diverse in its coverage of substantive areas, in its methodological approaches, as well as in its quality. Clearly, over two or so early decades of reading Foucault, nurses have applied his ideas to examine various facets of nursing practice (clinical, research, education, administration, regulation) across a range of settings (hospital, community and home care, psychiatric and mental health, corrections, university nursing programs, regulatory colleges, governmental agencies), as well as across a range of clinical populations. Moreover, a survey by Gastaldo and D. Holmes (1999) provided a sense of the breadth of application of Foucault's ideas in nursing. These authors reviewed 27 publications that explicitly draw on Foucault's work and were written by nurses in English (the bulk of the publications), Portuguese, and German. Gastaldo and Holmes pointed out a range of Foucauldian nursing critiques addressing the areas of nursing science, intensive and acute care, chronic renal illness, psychiatry and mental health, and the nurse–patient relationship. Buus and Hamilton (2016), in a systematic review of published studies of hospital documentation, such as nurses' records in patient charts, illustrated how Foucauldian concepts of power/knowledge and surveillance were used by researchers to make sense of nursing documentation practices.

Noticeably, this vast non-American postmodern and post-structural literature displayed certain similarities and overlaps with its American counterpart. For instance, the American nursing theory movement influenced disciplinary thinking well beyond the United States. Thus, the language of paradigms was not unique to American post-structural writings. Another example is how postmodern/post-structural feminism was handled in several papers in non-American nursing journals (e.g. Aranda, 2006; Aston et al., 2012; Crowe, 2000; Crowe & Alavi, 1999; Fahy, 1997; Francis, 2000; Huntington & Gilmour, 2001; Manias & Street, 2000;

Seibold, 2000). Some of these authors (e.g. Fahy, 1997; Huntington & Gilmour, 2001; Manias & Street, 2000, p. 58), despite their recognition of the tensions between certain feminist positions and postmodern criticisms, tended to preserve the "Self" of the essential subject and link Foucault to the emancipatory agenda rather unproblematically, similar to selected *ANS* papers examined in the previous chapter.

However, several nurse academics understood Foucault's insights sufficiently well to caution against specific (mis)apprehension of his work. This stream of publications discernible in non-American nursing literature (e.g. Cheek & Porter, 1997; Porter, 1998; Porter & O'Halloran, 2009) – but non-existent in the U.S. nursing discourse – comprised the critical appraisal of the suitability of Foucault's ideas for the discipline of nursing and pointed criticisms of selected nursing postmodern and post-structural scholarship. Recall that in *ANS* and some American "nursing knowledge" textbooks (Chinn & Kramer, 2011, 2015; Falk Rafael, 1997; Glass & Davis, 1998), the conflicting perspectives of German critical theorist Habermas and French post-structural theorist Foucault (and similarly conflicting perspectives of the second-wave feminists and Foucault), particularly their divergent conceptions of power and subjectivity, were combined rather cavalierly within the emancipatory agenda. These problematic uses of Foucault's ideas went unnoticed in the American theoretical discourse. In contrast, outside the United States, Irish nurse and sociologist Sam Porter, among others, articulately cautioned against such readings of Foucault. The problem with treating Foucault on a par with other critical theorists such as Weber, Marx, and radical feminists (most notably those challenging the medicalization of the female body) was directly addressed by Porter (Cheek & Porter, 1997). He rightly pointed out the dissolution of the subject in Foucault's theory: the very subject – autonomous and susceptible to empowerment – central to modernist-humanist critical theories. My specific interest in highlighting Porter's work is his warranted rejection of a simplistic fusing of Foucault with emancipatory/empowerment agenda, a common practice in "non-enclave" American nursing literature.[2]

Another risk of misapprehending Foucault's work is related to the conversion of postmodern and post-structural theory into qualitative methodology. Three nurse scholars with a particularly good grasp of Foucauldian nursing scholarship (Buus, 2005; Nelson, 2003; Traynor, 2003, 2006, 2013) have exposed serious issues related to this trend – a trend they observed across nursing literature in the 1990s to early 2000s. For one, these critics pointed out the practice of loading the front part of the research report with what those qualitative researchers believed should be a coherent account of "ontology-epistemology-method-validity criteria" while leaving the study findings under-theorized. The other issue was the severing of postmodern and post-structural "qualitative research method(ology)" from an ongoing exchange with relevant disciplines and thus with the impetus and theoretical tools these disciplinary traditions provide. Yet, as critics pointed out, these contemporary intellectual tools could benefit nursing research. They could assist researchers to theorize the "subjective" interview material within the social, political, and historical context – a move corresponding to the postmodern and post-structural de-centring of the metanarrative of human consciousness as the "Author" of its experience and "knowledge."

Non-American nurse scholars productively engaged with Foucauldian ideas during this period were some of the members of the *In Sickness and in Health* (*ISIH*) group. Trudy Rudge and her students, colleagues, and co-authors drew on a variety of social theory, often in the context of ethnographic and discourse-analytic studies (e.g. Rudge & D. Holmes, 2010). Christine Ceci, Kristine Bjorns-dottir, and Mary Ellen Purkis (Ceci, 2006; Ceci et al., 2012) led a program of empirical research informed by actor-network and practice theories and Fou-cault's insights. Their theoretically robust empirical studies of nursing practice informed by continental ideas (Ceci & Purkis, 2010; Ceci et al., 2012) moved to an interdisciplinary terrain and to high-ranking sociology journals. This partici-pation of nursing scholarship in larger scholarly debates attests to the quality of nursing work; it also demands high literacy from nurse educators to make such strong examples of nursing scholarship relatable for nursing students.

Other members of *ISIH* include Denise Gastaldo and Dave Holmes. Their names first appeared in *NI* in 1999 in "Foucault and Nursing: A History of the Present" (Gastaldo & Holmes, 1999) and in *JAN* in 2002 in "Nursing as Means of Governmentality" (Holmes & Gastaldo, 2002). Holmes, professor of nursing from the University of Ottawa, is editor of the bilingual journal *Aporia*, launched in 2009. His publications and those of several of his doctoral students, mentees, and/or colleagues – Perron, O'Byrne, McCabe, Gagnon, Jacob, St-Pierre, and others (e.g. Holmes et al., 2012, 2014) – showed a lively and often provocative use of Foucault's ideas. Holmes's writings have generated heated polemics in nurs-ing literature and beyond (e.g. Porter & O'Halloran, 2009, 2010; Sandelowski, 2003). Noteworthy too, the kind of postmodern and post-structural scholarship exemplified by these Canadian authors, unlike their earlier Australian and Brit-ish counterparts, did not usually take as their intellectual backdrop, or as their opponent, American nursing theory. On the contrary, collaborative projects were united by the "emancipatory praxis" rubric (Kagan et al., 2014).

After 2010, the post-structural/Foucauldian nursing scene has been changing and somewhat shrinking. Particularly, the number of relevant articles dropped markedly in *JAN* that in the past led in publishing this kind of work. Simulta-neously, however, other nursing journals such as those from Scandinavia and especially Brazil published more Foucault-informed studies. Danish scholars (e.g. Frederiksen & Beedholm, 2017) have taken up Foucault's ideas in a fruitful way. Up to the date of writing, *Aporia*, *Nursing Inquiry*, and to a lesser degree *Nursing Philosophy*, have remained primary venues for French-theoretical scholarship.[3]

From this overview, I now turn to specifics to provide a theoretical background for the notion of nurse–patient relationships, the topic pursued by the first of my two exemplars of Foucauldian scholarship: Carl May.

Theorizing Nurse–Patient Relationships

Although nurse–patient interaction and nurse–patient relationships are highly relevant both as the very fabric of clinical nursing practice and a legitimate topic of disciplinary study, as well as the site where, from a Foucauldian perspective, power manifests and subjectivities are fabricated, the American nursing literature that explicitly cited postmodern and post-structural ideas in the 1990s and the 2000s had (with rare exception) directed its attention elsewhere, forgoing the study of nurse–patient interactions and nurse–patient relationships.[4] From 62 articles informed by postmodern and post-structural writings and authored by American nurses and/or published in American nursing periodicals (compiled in Table A1), only 2 – by Gadow (1999/2009) and Benner (2004) – referred to, or attempted to theorize, the nurse–patient encounter.

Sally Gadow (1999/2009), in her philosophical discussion of the "postmodern turn in nursing ethics," expressed an important idea about how the notion of meaning was understood by contemporary social theorists who wrote about human life in postmodern times. The notion of meaning itself is not guaranteed in the postmodern world. "Ethically, we are on our own, without a metaphysical warrant from either religion or reason" (Gadow, 1999/2009, p. 576). The implication of this insight for nursing practice, Gadow wrote, is that the meaning of a patient's illness or meanings of a nurse–patient encounter are not a priori truths that the nurse will access either in a detached, "objective" way, or a hermeneutic, "subjective" manner. Rather, these meanings are contingent on relational narrative; that is, the selves of the nurse and the patient do not pre-exist their encounter but arise in the process (Gadow, 1999/2009).

Although the term *relational* is common in contemporary nursing academic discourse, Gadow's (1999/2009) article is perhaps a rare example hinting at the key feature of relationality in a postmodern sense – the disappearance of the humanistic subject as the autonomous self-identical actor. Yet it is precisely this humanistic conception of the nurse and the patient that implicitly or explicitly grounds the entire canon of American nursing theory. Even occasional insertions of Gadow's paper in past editions of American anthologies of theoretical and metatheoretical nursing work (such as Cody, 2006; Kenney, 2002; Reed & Shearer, 2009) did not seem to trigger any reconsideration of the notion of the humanistic subject in American nursing theory literature including its postmodern and post-structural variety.[5]

Another American scholar, Patricia Benner (2004), selectively cited Foucault in the context of her writing about the ethics of nurse–patient encounters but did not go as far as to analyse nursing practice in light of Foucault's ideas on power and subjectivity. Instead, she limited Foucault's input within her critique of the dehumanizing clinical gaze of medicine, while praising nurses' role in retrieving "the person" behind the patient through nurses' humanizing language. This approach, according to a Canadian Foucauldian nurse scholar, Purkis (1994, 2013; Purkis & Bjornsdottir, 2006), failed to recognize the nurse–patient encounter as a contentious site of power. Benner's position drawing on Foucault's critique of the clinical gaze in relation to medicine was not new; it was shared across a range of theoretical perspectives in the discipline. For Benner, as for many other nurse theorists, a rejection of the reductionist medical gaze served to elevate the humanizing and holistic nurse–patient relationship as an aspiration for nursing practice. In contrast, a well-argued and pioneering example of non-American scholarship presented in the following demonstrates a different kind of Foucauldian analysis of nurse–patient relationships and nurse–patient interaction.

In the 1990s, nursing and sociology journals published a series of papers by a British social scientist, Carl May, based on his doctoral study of bedside nursing practice. The study involved observations of nursing practice on acute-care wards in a Scottish hospital and interviews with nurses working there with terminally ill patients. May draws skilfully on Foucault's work to theorize nurse–patient interaction and relationships.[6]

May (1990) begins with examining how nurses tended to conceptualize nurse–patient relationships and/or interaction in their empirical studies of and theoretical writings about nursing practice. For his analysis, May divides selected literature into two types based on the researchers' conception of nurse–patient interaction and nurse–patient relationships: technocratic or contextual. In studies of the first type, researchers conceptualize nurse–patient interaction as the communicative action controlled by the individual nurse. The nurse is depicted as being able, by following a prescribed set of steps, to achieve a desired goal in the nurse–patient interaction. May calls this type of theoretical attitude of the researcher *technocratic* because it directs attention to the technical aspects of the interaction (such as its duration as well as the nurses' immediate behaviour and linguistic strategies to manage patient encounters). Findings of these empirical studies consistently demonstrate the brevity and task orientation of nurse–patient interaction as well as nurses' conversational tactics to maintain control over verbal interaction. Researchers, who declared their belief in the importance of interpersonal relations between nurses and patients, explain these somewhat disillusioning findings by focusing solely on the dyadic encounter between nurse and patient: Nurses' negative stereotyping of their patients or nurses' self-defence against occupational stress are responsible for the inadequate quality of nurse–patient interaction. (It is important to notice that May does not want to minimize the significance of these phenomena in nursing practice; his aim is to contrast this technocratic outlook commonly employed in research with what he calls contextual perspective.) The technocratic outlook presupposes considerable autonomy of the nurse, much exceeding that which nurses can reasonably exercise in their practice. May locates this conception of nurse–patient interactions in "nursing theory" that delineates what practice *should* be like and that influences nursing education and research. May is not explicit about the kind of "nursing theory," but he likely alludes to the theoretical prescriptions of nursing process and nursing diagnosis exported from the United States and implemented throughout the U.K. hospitals in the 1980s.

This technocratic attitude of researchers to nurse–patient interaction is contrasted by May (1990) with the *contextual* attitude to nurse–patient interaction. Rooted in social and social psychological theory, this approach recognizes the fundamentally social nature of the interaction. In May's words, the nurse–patient interaction is constituted within an organizational context and the occupational cultures of nurses and others on the ward. Dyadic interaction is an outcome of its social organization. In other words, the nurse–patient interaction/relationship is an example of a social, collective accomplishment.[7]

May (1990) recognizes that *both* groups of researchers, technocratic and contextual, are motivated by a similar desire to enhance nurse–patient relationships, to move them away from the "body parts that need fixing" type of encounter to a more humane process. What, however, is different are the *effects* produced by writing (about) nursing practice in those particular ways. The very ability of the nurse to engage in a meaningful relationship with the patient is socially organized: determined by organizational context. But the technocratic attitude of some nursing theory, focused on the individuated action, does not allow this understanding to emerge. May finds the contextual approach to the study of nurse–patient relationships more useful than the technocratic one. Specifically, he proposes the value of inductive theorizing rooted in the sociological perspective of symbolic interactionism and perhaps informed by Foucault's concepts.

Writing about nurse–patient relationships, May (1990) alludes to another analytical line that he develops more fully in his other publications – the importance attached to the nurse–patient relationship in contemporary nursing. Connected to nursing's professionalizing efforts, this emphasis on nurse–patient relationships signifies a break with nursing's previous narrow focus on the physiological factors, a focus aligned with the domain of medicine. It is clear from May's tone, however, that he is far from romanticizing nursing's professional ideology that "fabricates" a new nurse–patient relationship (May, 1990, p. 311). Bringing Foucault's notion of power/knowledge to bear on his analysis, May (1990) points out the process of the "reconstitution of patients 'needs' and psychosocial problems, through which a technical vocabulary emerges containing new signs and symptoms" (p. 312).

May identifies this professional ideology as the discourse of holism dominating American nursing theory. The shift towards holism was part of a program of nursing professional differentiation from medicine and closure from incursions by other allied health occupations (May & Fleming, 1997). American academic nurse leaders envisioned the professionalization of nursing as depending on a construction of "unique" knowledge – most notably, in the form of holistic nursing theory – as differentiated from biomedicine (May & Purkis, 1995). The strictly biomedical way to "apprehend the patient" (May, 1992a, p. 589) as a biological entity was augmented by new techniques of individualization and surveillance to apprehend the patient as a psychosocial entity. Thus, May problematizes the holistic nurse–patient relationship as a site of production of the patient's "real" self.

May (1992a) analyses holistic practice, or individualized attention to the whole person – a discourse that in nursing literature carries an unquestionably positive and desirable connotation – in light of Foucault's ideas about the processes of subjectification as a contemporary mechanism of power in health care institutions. In the context of individualized holistic care, the patient is encouraged to become an "experiencing" subject, to produce and disclose her inner dispositions and identity. A "talk" between a nurse and a patient is a crucial site for the production of confessing subjectivities. Following Foucault, May (1992a) writes,

> Power is not an objective phenomenon, but rather a quality of the discourses and practices activated with social relationships, and as such exists only in the moment of its exercise. . . . Foucault insists on the importance and vitality of pastoral power as a quality of the relationship between institutions which rely on surveillance and their subjects.
>
> (p. 596)

A nursing ideal of individualized care is to be achieved through "talk" in the context of the nurse–patient relationship, which retrieves a patient's authentic self by inviting the patient to account for her social and psychological "problems" (May, 1995a). However, May refuses to accept a commonsensical explanation for this shift towards individualized holistic nursing. Instead, he interprets psychosocial nursing care as "surveillance, or monitoring, of the intimate disposition of the subject [which] is a key mode of exercizing power" (May, 1995a, p. 557) in nursing practice.

Taking into consideration the actualities of the social organization of nursing practice, May (1995b) points out the pragmatic issues with the holistic model of nursing care – in particular the unreasonable expectation that nurses produce "authentic relationships" with patients. Professional discourses, most notably nursing theory, although not meant to speak to the empirical realities of practice, nevertheless place demands on nurses' conduct. Nursing theory (May, 1995b, cites Newman and Parse) is a sophisticated conceptual apparatus imposing implicit prescriptions for, and supplying understandings of, nurse–patient encounters in the context of increased "individualization" of care.

May agrees that individualized care based on "knowing the patient" often provides an ethical base for humane provision of health services (May, 1992b, p. 482). However, he wants to destabilize the romantic vision of the nurse–patient relationship said to provide access to such "knowledge." The patient is "known" through the deployment of the clinical gaze, both medical *and* nursing, which is how power manifests. Further, May points out some unacknowledged practical obstacles to nurses' *work* of producing "good" personal relationships with patients. On the one hand, nurses themselves can resist attempts to "know" patients. On the other hand, a patient can remain silent when a nurse asks, *What kind of person are you?*, thus denying the nurse's legitimacy to ask such a question. May argues that those nurses theorizing the nurse–patient relationship need to consider the practical problems that are negotiated – by both nurses and their patients – when nurses attempt to get to "know" their patients (May, 1992b).

In summary, this example of May's work of theorizing nurse–patient relationships through the lens of Foucault's concepts denaturalizes a conception of this relationship as a power-free encounter controlled solely by the nurse's benevolent intent and valorized in the trope of "knowing the patient." Power manifests through the nurse's gaze, surveillance, "talk," and through the patient's resistance to legitimate the nurse's gesture to retrieve the "whole," authentic subject of the patient.

I would like to conclude this first case of non-American post-structural scholarship by highlighting one of its key – but perhaps not immediately obvious – characteristics that creates an even sharper contrast with the handling of post-structural theory in the American nursing disciplinary matrix. An important *condition of possibility* for the sophisticated application of Foucault's ideas in May's and other writings lies in the authors' conception of nursing practice as a *social* activity. Whereas American nursing theory often treats nursing as ahistorical, acontextual, and comprised of individuated intentions and acts, May and other authors are dexterous with conceptual tools developed in the social sciences such as sociology, which can produce interesting and rigorous understandings of nursing. Many great Australian, British, and Canadian examples of postmodern and post-structural nursing theorizing (e.g. compiled in Table A3), presuppose nursing as socially and historically contingent practices – an understanding lacking in the American nursing theory counterparts.

Nurse scholars' appreciation of the relevance of contemporary social theory for understanding nursing practice, or, at the very least, their assumption that nursing is historically and socially contingent, provides fertile soil for postmodern and post-structural nursing scholarship, as is evident in many non-American examples *and* a few American ones (e.g. by David Allen, Drevdahl, Liaschenko, Sandelowski, Thompson). On the other hand, simply claiming some tenuous link to one or another sociological perspective among "paradigmatic origins" (e.g. Meleis, 2007, p. 336) of a nursing theory neither guarantees a rigorous application of this sociological perspective nor provides an adequate "bridge" for the nursing theory to consequently be revised in light of revisions that the claimed sociological perspective undergoes in its home discipline.

A relevant example in the context of my discussion of nurse–patient interaction can be drawn from Afaf Meleis's impressive monograph *Theoretical Nursing: Development and Progress* (1997, 2007). Meleis (1997, 2007) classified selected American nursing theories as belonging to the "interaction school of thought" – based on nurse theorists' view of nursing "as supporting and promoting interactions with patients" (Meleis, 1997, p. 114). She identified the sociological perspectives of systems theory and symbolic interactionism as having influenced these nursing works. However, on a closer examination, these nursing theories have been criticized by a German nurse scholar, Wied (2006), as eclectic and vague in their application of sociological concepts of systems and interactions, as failing to consider the ongoing developments in sociology and, importantly, as having lost a *sociological* angle, that is, an assumption of, as well as the implications flowing from, the socialness of nursing practice and nurse–patient interaction. Thus, the supposedly interaction-focused (in the sociological sense) nursing theories of Peplau and King, in fact present an unacknowledged individual-focused bias, which encourages a humanistic view of nurse–patient interaction as an unmediated exchange of two or more autonomous consciousnesses (Wied, 2006).

This imprecision and the reification of sociological concepts in American nursing theories originally informed by sociological perspectives and a lack of exchange between this body of nursing scholarship and subsequent developments and debates in the social sciences, may provide a clue to the source of the pervasive cumulative style of American treatises on "nursing knowledge" (including Meleis's texts). In this style, new social-theoretical and philosophical ideas are enthusiastically added to the old nursing disciplinary matrix rather than used to pry this matrix open for critical interrogation. A list of long-running editions of nursing theory textbooks in Table A2 provides several examples of such treatment of postmodern and post-structural ideas.

The Holistic Nurse Through a Historical Lens

Sioban Nelson is a nurse historian, whose book *A Genealogy of Care of the Sick: Nursing, Holism, and Pious Practice* (2000) offers an explanation for the immense popularity of spiritual concerns in contemporary professional (and what is considered secularized) nursing, concerns captured in the emphasis on holism and humanism present in much nursing theory. I will summarize Nelson's thesis before moving on to connect her argument with the topic of my study.

How has the figure of the holistic nurse come to dominate the discursive field of nursing in the second half of the 20th century, especially in American theoretical literature? What are we to make of a widespread pedagogy that demands nursing students "listen" to patients' calls for spiritual healing and promote their spiritual growth, on the one hand, and to look inward and work on their own spiritual resources in a quest for self-actualization, on the other? Why have the humanistic ideals of American nurse theorists gained a widespread acceptance? Nelson poses these questions and looks for answers in a 2,000-year-old history of the care of the sick in the West. This long look enables her to challenge the conventional historical account of modern professional nursing. According to the latter, secular nursing practice emerging in the second half of the 19th century has shed the legacies of the religious nursing orders, most notably the Christian imperative of *agape* or "love of strangers" (Nelson, 2000, pp. 8–9). Moreover, in this conventional depiction, the contemporary humanist/holistic nurse appears as the pinnacle of nursing's professional evolution. It is this depiction that troubles Nelson.

Aided by the theoretical notions of *technologies of the self* from Foucault (Nelson, 2000, pp. 49–50) along with *habitus* and *personae* from Marcel Mauss (pp. 5–7), Nelson argues that contemporary nursing's interest in spiritual concerns is part of the Christian ethos that founded the care of the sick throughout two millennia. The term *ethos* denotes sets of practices, ways of relating to oneself, techniques of working on oneself, or self-culture (Pierre Hadot's notion of *askesis*; Nelson, 2000, p. 7). *Christian ethos* refers to ways to transform oneself into the instrument of God. As a two-way road, Christian ethos works to redeem the soul of the cared for while accruing virtue for the soul of the carer. No doubt, the ways in which this Christian ethos manifests have changed over time, and no linear, integrated history of those processes can be told. One of the most obvious shifts is the rejection of religious vocabulary; in Nelson's view, however, this shift should not mask the continuity of the essentially Christian concern for the souls of the sick, "evident in both the theoreticians' schemata and the practice manuals alike" (pp. 4–5). In contemporary nursing, the "self-evident" ethical holistic (and spiritual) ideal is embodied by the "single . . . persona – the humanistic nurse" (p. 6). Challenging the self-evident nature of such a belief, Nelson insists that this professional persona with her holistic ethical deportment is a specialized product of the *habitus* of nursing, "comprised of a complex of habitual modes of thought, habits of body and soul, plus their modes of transmission and relation to specific social settings" (p. 5). So rather than viewing the holistic-humanistic imperative as a high point in the evolution of the secular nursing profession, Nelson proposes another answer to the question she raised.

According to Nelson's (2000) analysis, the holistic ethos of nursing reflects an abiding attempt to instil a particular ethical deportment (through self-transformation techniques) into nurse recruits: to *train* today's nurses in the (Christian) ethos of *agape* in a liberal academy that otherwise is mostly concerned with knowledge and technical skills. The prominence of holistic-humanistic American nursing theory owes much to the anxiety-generating idea that nursing will be reduced to "mere technical knowledge and skills" if academic nursing preparation does not instil caring as an unquestioned virtue, the value of the patient's and nurse's self-transcendence, a search for meaning, and spiritual growth. Nelson suggests that nursing theory be viewed as a response to a serious concern, even a dread; that nursing, the *vocation* of care for the sick, can be conceived as only a technical skill; that a nurse, for example, can come to regard it solely as a means of financial sustenance.

Once American nursing moved to the liberal academy after World War II and nursing practice in hospitals was increasingly technologized, nurse scholars (in what is commonly depicted as a counter-dehumanizing effort) began to articulate the body of holistic nursing science based on a loosely defined "humanist philosophy." Nelson cites the themes of interpersonal human relations, the caring moment, patient-centredness, and the wholeness of the person (both patient and nurse). From the 1960s, such an emphasis on humanistic values has been a crucial part of professional nursing's self-image. The figure of a holistic nurse – "a foil for the impersonal and segmented medical gaze" (p. 11) who views the human being as an irreducible entity needed to be rescued from the uncaring environment – is an aspiration to be held out to nursing students and for them to grasp. One of the curricular instruments to achieve a desired nursing ethos is reflective journaling, which, Nelson argues, functions as a new technology of the self.

But there is more to Nelson's argument than the intent to link the holistic ethos of secular nursing to the old Christian imperative of agape and to complicate the naturalized humanistic, patient-centred philosophy of nursing. Perhaps what she finds the most irksome throughout the holistic-humanistic literature is the "colonization" of the influential nursing academic texts by highly idealized and transcendent accounts of nursing practice. These accounts, Nelson argues, valorize the holistic nurse – one for whom agape becomes nothing less than a way of life – who continually works on oneself to achieve spiritual immediacy with her clients. Valorizing the ideal of the "whole" nurse and her spiritual ethos, these accounts elide mundane depictions of nurses' daily and nightly realities and mask the fact that not all nurses and patients strive for "transcendent caring moments."

What does all this have to do with my interest in nurses' receptivity to continental philosophy? In responding to this question, I would like to start by imparting two points pertinent to my analysis. First, both Nelson's (2000) and Risjord's (2010) analyses offer something like a breakthrough in our understanding of American theoretical nursing writings. And these two analyses valuably complement each other. Comprising the body of a unique nursing science, several well-known works of American nurse theorists are collectively known as holistic and humanistic. As described before, Nelson examines the colonization of nursing's academic field by themes of holism and humanism in American nursing theory. A set of writings examined by Nelson partially overlaps with those examined by Risjord (e.g. Carper, Chinn and Kramer, King, Meleis, Neuman, Reed). But if Risjord looked at the tropes of science and structure of theory from a perspective of the philosophy of science (an appropriate move considering that nurse theorists regard their work as scientific and cite philosophers of science), Nelson read the body of texts for their ideological, professional content. Risjord studied "the packaging" (and that's why he took care to distinguish the early writings by Peplau, V. Henderson, and Wiedenbach as "philosophies" in a colloquial sense from later nursing theory that aspired to the status of "science"). Nelson examined the message, the valorization of the ethical ethos of a holistic-humanistic nurse. And here I come to the second point, crucial to the case I am making.

I suggest that nurses do not (necessarily) read nursing theory as science; many of them simply do not have the philosophy of science background essential to understand and evaluate nursing theory *as* scientific theory. Nurse educators read American theory as poetry (Tschanz, 2005, p. 110); "beyond and beneath the words," in the sense of going beyond specific words to look for resonances with one's emotions, memories, and thoughts (Doane &Varcoe, 2005, p. 108); ideology; "religion of nursing" (Dickoff & James, 1971/1997, p. 59); "nonrealist nursing ontologies" (Flaming, 2004); and "philosophizing" in a colloquial sense of the term (Thorne, 2014, p. 81). If we agree with this statement, then Nelson's analysis clarifies how nursing audiences (educators, scholars, students, and perhaps some practitioners in clinical settings) read American nursing theory, what they find there, and why they value it: as a powerful technique to cultivate ethical deportment in nursing students. This might be a legitimate purpose, had it not been for some thorny issues. First, the edifying, ideological purpose of nursing theory is neither explicitly acknowledged nor evaluated as the best possible strategy to teach nursing students moral values of caring and empathy. (Another option might be "nursing humanities," i.e., liberal arts education based on great novels or quality education in nursing history.) Second, since the 1970s the voluminous and growing body of nursing theory writings has strongly established itself in the discipline, especially in the United States and Canada, as an epistemological field of "nursing knowledge" constituting an appealing and accessible model for replication (in fact, an outdated scientific model as Risjord demonstrated) and legitimating what counts as worthy intellectual endeavour and product. My book surfaces the problematic influence of this American intellectual matrix on nurses. The central influence is that nurses, especially nursing students, may be discouraged from using contemporary continental philosophy and social theory because they are considered to be borrowed, anti-humanist, and androcentric. I claim that the central issue related to the American discourse of "nursing knowledge" is that it produces invisibility and unintelligibility of practices of theorizing in the discipline of nursing based on contemporary interdisciplinary social philosophy and theory, *as these are practiced in the humanities and the social sciences.*

If Risjord's (2010) analysis suggests that proper nursing theory has been (mis)conceived by many nurse scholars particularly in the United States as having an axiomatic structure, lending itself to one of the logical levels, linked to the nursing metaparadigm, and preferably not borrowed, then Nelson's (2000) work, in a complementary manner, suggests that proper nursing theory has been (mis)conceived as obliged to carry an ideological, edifying message. In this image, nursing theorizing should capture the holistic, spiritual, humanistic, and transcendent aspects – all which aids in the process of introspection and self-transformation, always with a twin goal to help the client in a process of transcendence. It is not a big leap to speculate that if a nurse reader looks only for such a message, chances are much continental and social theoretical scholarship will be overlooked as (ir)relevant nursing knowledge. I indicated in Chapter 2 that certain strands of continental thought fit with this agenda, and thus nursing has been more receptive to those. The challenge, however, is that the most radical kinds of continental thought, what in North America has been dubbed "French theory" (Cusset, 2008) but not limited to it, not only is a poor fit with humanist ideology but undermines its assumptions. We have seen precisely this in Nelson's study that unravels the "whole" nurse with the aid of the French theoretical toolbox.

Concluding Thoughts

Non-American postmodern, post-structural, and Foucauldian scholarship published in the 1990s to the 2010s is vast in quantity and uneven in quality. I sketched only its contours and pointed out noticeable features. Overall, applications of French theory generated outside of the American disciplinary matrix can be summarized with the metaphor *via negativa:*[8]

- They do not deploy the discourse of nursing science or unique nursing theory.
- They do not seek to locate their projects within the "structure of disciplinary knowledge."
- They do not seek to protect this structure from being unravelled by postmodern and post-structural conceptions of meaning and language.
- They do not seek to preserve the assumptions of "nursing theory" from being unravelled by the post-humanist conceptions of power and subjectivity.

- They do not (or do not necessarily) seek to legitimate nursing knowledge by recourse to the binaries of nursing/medicine, care/cure, or postmodern research/positivist scientific method.
- They do not subsume Foucault under the emancipatory agenda (and treat such attempts with caution).
- They are not wary of "borrowed" theory (such as continental philosophy, sociology and anthropology, history) but embrace these influences as necessary for theoretical rigour in the discipline of nursing.

This summary of features not present in writings generated outside of the American nursing matrix exposes a sharp contrast between some of the best examples of Australian, British, and Canadian postmodern and post-structural nursing scholarship (and the small number of works by the enclave nurses in the United States) and their American nursing theory counterpart where these features inhere. This summary also lays bare elements of the "unique nursing science" – those elements mightily contributing to the continuing invisibility and unintelligibility of postmodern and post-structural continental philosophy and non-American postmodern/post-structural scholarship in American nursing literature.

In the latter part of the chapter, I showcased two prominent examples of pioneering Foucauldian scholarship. These examples by Carl May and Sioban Nelson problematized a widely accepted holistic ideal as a superior ethical stance (Nelson) and as a model of practice that valorizes "knowing the patient" as an egalitarian and self-evident configuration of the nurse–patient relationship (May). As far as I can tell, these (non-American) criticisms of the theoretical holistic movement were invisible in American nursing literature at least into the second decade of the 21st century: I have not encountered citations to their work summarized in this chapter in any of the American anthologies or surveys of "nursing theory and nursing knowledge" I reviewed (Tables A1 and A2).[9]

Notes

1 As discussed earlier, in American nursing literature, postmodern and post-structural continental philosophical critiques of nursing theory and/or methodological discussions have been undertaken by the enclave scholars, by some American nurses with a humanities background (e.g. Liaschenko and Sandelowski), and by non-nurses in one interdisciplinary and international collection on nursing theory (Kim & Kollak, 2006).

2 Similarly, several other non-American nurse authors pointed out the tensive relationship between Foucault's stance and emancipatory projects (Aranda, 2006; Rolfe, 2000, p. 155; Traynor, 1997).

3 A CINAHL search in March 2022 using variations of keywords *postmodernism*, *post-structuralism*, or *Foucault* in All Text, for articles published in English from January 2011 to the end of 2021, produced the following numbers of hits in relevant nursing journals:

> *Aporia* (editor Dave Holmes) 45; *Nursing Inquiry* 40; *Journal of Nursing ufpe / revista de enfermagem ufpe* 34 and five other Brazilian journals between 9–30 each; *Scandinavian Journal of Caring Sciences* 30; *Nursing Philosophy* 28; *Journal of Clinical Nursing* 22; *Qualitative Health Research* 20; *Journal of Advanced Nursing*, *Nursing Ethics*, and other journals 8 or fewer each.

4 A few American nurses not pursuing a postmodern/post-structural theoretical route (most notably Liaschenko, 1997, and Lowenberg, 1995, 2003) have analysed the nurse–patient relationship from other theoretical perspectives.

5 Likely, the opposite was the case. Writing style and emphases in Gadow's work (e.g. 2000) are highly reminiscent of the era of English romanticism with its deep divide between science and poetry (Paley, 2004), and thus her work lent itself to be received as another example of anti-science, humanistic nursing theory. Interestingly, Nelson (2000) critiqued Gadow's work as representative of the American holistic nursing theory movement. However, Nelson (2000, p. 212) referred to Gadow's early writings on existential advocacy and clinical subjectivity, not to Gadow's paper I examined.

6 Although May is not a nurse, my rationale for focusing on his work includes the following: (a) it is the *earliest* example of Foucault-based analysis of nursing practice published in nursing journals with international circulation, *Journal of Advanced Nursing* and *International Journal of Nursing Studies*; (b) the author's social scientific background facilitates his well-informed reading of Foucault's work, a characteristic that cannot be assumed in all nursing writings; (c) the focus of his research is nursing practice – a topic nearly absent in American nursing theoretical literature; and (d) his work avoids crude anti-science rhetoric that plagues many postmodern and post-structural nursing writings.

7 May acknowledges that even though this understanding of nurse–patient interaction moves away from the dyadic view, it still remains within the bounds of local context, for example, negotiations among different professional groups and patients. May is somewhat vague on this point. I speculate that what he has in mind is another sociological perspective, the so-called macro perspective, which transcends both a micro-level of the dyad *and* a meso-level of organizational context and instead looks at the economic conditions. Debates among the proponents of these differing perspectives in sociology are well documented (e.g. Porter, 1998).

8 I thank Dr. Madeline Walker for offering this term.

9 On the other hand, Margarete Sandelowski (1998, 2002, Barnard & Sandelowski, 2001), who is not recognized as a "theorist" by the nursing canon despite her perceptive theoretical writings on technology, did cite May's work and some Australian nurses who theorize in a postmodern vein. Indeed, Sandelowski's writings on technology are so thoroughly postmodern in spirit (she avoids the label *postmodernism* while favouring posthuman feminist or "cyborg feminist" literature) – that is, dismantling the binary oppositions – that her work too remains unintelligible within the American disciplinary matrix.

References

Aranda, K. (2006). Postmodern feminist perspectives and nursing research: A passionately interested form of inquiry. *Nursing Inquiry, 13*(2), 135–143.

Aston, M., Price, S., Kirk, S. L., & Penney, T. (2012). More than meets the eye. Feminist poststructuralism as a lens towards understanding obesity. *Journal of Advanced Nursing, 68*(5), 1187–1194.

Barnard, A., & Sandelowski, M. (2001). Technology and humane nursing care: (Ir)reconcilable or invented difference. *Journal of Advanced Nursing, 34*(3), 367–375.

Benner, P. (2004). Seeing the person beyond the disease. *American Journal of Critical Care, 13*(1), 75–78.

Buus, N. (2005). Nursing scholars appropriating new methods: The use of discourse analysis in scholarly nursing journals 1996–2003. *Nursing Inquiry, 12*(1), 27–33.

Buus, N., & Hamilton, B. E. (2016). Social science and linguistic text analysis of nurses' records: A systematic review and critique. *Nursing Inquiry, 23*(1), 64–77.

Ceci, C. (2006). "What she says she needs doesn't make a lot of sense": Seeing and knowing in a field study of home-care case management. *Nursing Philosophy, 7,* 90–99.

Ceci, C. (2012). "To work out what works best": What is good care in home care. In C. Ceci, M. E. Purkis, & K. Björnsdóttir (Eds.), *Perspectives on care at home for older people* (pp. 81–100). Routledge.

Ceci, C., & Purkis, M. E. (2010). Implications of an epistemological vision: Knowing what to do in home health care. In C. Patton (Ed.), *Rebirth of the clinic: Places and agents in contemporary health care* (pp. 17–37). University of Minnesota Press.

Chapman, G. (1988). Reporting therapeutic discourse in a therapeutic community. *Journal of Advanced Nursing, 13*(2), 255–264.

Cheek, J., & Porter, S. (1997). Reviewing Foucault: Possibilities and problems for nursing and health care. *Nursing Inquiry, 4*(2), 108–119.

Chinn, P. L., & Kramer, M. K. (2011). *Integrated theory and knowledge development in nursing* (8th ed.). Elsevier Mosby.

Chinn, P. L., & Kramer, M. K. (2015). *Knowledge development in nursing: Theory and process* (9th ed.). Elsevier Health Sciences.

Cody, W. K. (Ed.). (2006). *Philosophical and theoretical perspectives for advanced nursing practice* (4th ed.). Jones and Bartlett Publishers.

Crowe, M. (2000). The nurse–patient relationship: A consideration of its discursive context. *Journal of Advanced Nursing, 31*(4), 962–967.

Crowe, M., & Alavi, C. (1999). Mad talk: Attending to the language of distress. *Nursing Inquiry, 6*(1), 26–33.

Cusset, F. (2008). *French theory: How Foucault, Derrida, Deleuze, & Co. transformed the intellectual life of the United States* (J. Fort, Trans.). University of Minnesota Press.

Dickoff, J., & James, P. (1997). Clarity to what end? In L. H. Nicoll (Ed.), *Perspectives on nursing theory* (3rd ed., pp. 55–61). Lippincott. (Original work published in *Nursing Research, 20*(6), 499–502, in 1971)

Doane, G. H., & Varcoe, C. (2005). *Family nursing as relational inquiry: Developing health-promoting practice.* Lippincott Williams & Wilkins.

Dzurec, L. (1989). The necessity for and evolution of multiple paradigms for nursing research: A poststructuralist perspective. *Advances in Nursing Science, 11*(4), 69–77.

Fahy, K. (1997). Postmodern feminist emancipatory research: Is it an oxymoron? *Nursing Inquiry, 4*(1), 27–33.

Falk Rafael, A. R. (1997). Advocacy oral history: A research methodology for social activism in nursing. *Advances in Nursing Science, 20*(2), 32–44.

Flaming, D. (2004). Nursing theories as nursing ontologies. *Nursing Philosophy, 5*(3), 224–229.

Francis, B. (2000). Poststructuralism and nursing: Uncomfortable bedfellows? *Nursing Inquiry, 7*(1), 20–28.

Frederiksen, K., & Beedholm, K. (2017). Foucault, social theory and nursing research: A critique. In M. Lipscomb (Ed.), *Social theory and nursing* (pp. 119–133). Routledge.

Gadow, S. (2000). Philosophy as falling: Aiming for grace. *Nursing Philosophy, 1*(2), 89–97.

Gadow, S. (2009). Relational narrative: The postmodern turn in nursing ethics. In P. G. Reed & N. B. C. Shearer (Eds.), *Perspectives on nursing theory* (5th ed., pp. 571–580). (Original work published in *Scholarly Inquiry for Nursing Practice, 13*(1), 57–70, in 1999)

Gastaldo, D., & Holmes, D. (1999). Foucault and nursing: A history of the present. *Nursing Inquiry, 6*(4), 231–240.

Glass, N., & Davis, K. (1998). An emancipatory impulse: A feminist postmodern integrated turning point in nursing research. *Advances in Nursing Science, 21*(1), 43–52.

Holmes, D., & Gastaldo, D. (2002). Nursing as means of governmentality. *Journal of Advanced Nursing, 38*(6), 557–565.

Holmes, D., Jacob, J. D., & Perron, A. (Eds.). (2014). *Power and the psychiatric apparatus: Repression, transformation, and assistance.* Ashgate.

Holmes, D., Rudge, T., & Perron, A. (Eds.). (2012). *(Re)thinking violence in healthcare: A critical perspective.* Ashgate.

Huntington, A., & Gilmour, J. (2001). Re-thinking representations, re-writing nursing texts: Possibilities through feminist and Foucauldian thought. *Journal of Advanced Nursing, 35*(6), 902–908.

Kagan, P. N., Smith, M. C., & Chinn, P. L. (Eds.). (2014). *Philosophies and practices of emancipatory nursing: Social justice as praxis.* Routledge.

Kenney, J. W. (Ed.). (2002). *Philosophical and theoretical perspectives for advanced nursing practice* (3rd ed.). Jones and Bartlett Publishers.

Kim, H. S., & Kollak, I. (Eds.). (2006). *Nursing theories: Conceptual and philosophical foundations* (2nd ed.). Springer Publishing Company.

Lees, G., Richman, J., Salauroo, M., & Warden, S. (1987). Quality assurance: Is it professional insurance? *Journal of Advanced Nursing, 12*(6), 719–727.

Liaschenko, J. (1997). Ethics and the geography of the nurse–patient relationship: Spatial vulnerabilities and gendered space. *Scholarly Inquiry for Nursing Practice, 11*(1), 45–59.

Lowenberg, J. S. (1995). Response to "The configuration of nurse–patient relationships: A critical view." *Scholarly Inquiry for Nursing Practice, 9*(4), 297–301.

Lowenberg, J. S. (2003). The nurse–client relationship in a stress management clinic. *Holistic Nursing Practice, 17*(2), 99–109.

Manias, E., & Street, A. (2000). Possibilities for critical social theory and Foucault's work: A toolbox approach. *Nursing Inquiry, 7*(1), 50–60.

May, C. R. (1990). Research on nurse–patient relationships: Problems of theory, problems of practice. *Journal of Advanced Nursing, 15*(3), 307–315.

May, C. R. (1992a). Individual care – power and subjectivity in therapeutic relationships. *Sociology, 26*(4), 589–602.

May, C. R. (1992b). Nursing work, nurses' knowledge, and the subjectification of the patient. *Sociology of Health and Illness, 14*(4), 472–487.

May, C. R. (1995a). "To call it work somehow demeans it": The social construction of talk in the care of terminally ill patients. *Journal of Advanced Nursing, 22*(3), 556–561.

May, C. R. (1995b). Patient autonomy and the politics of professional relationships. *Journal of Advanced Nursing, 21*(1), 83–87.

May, C. R., & Fleming, C. (1997). The professional imagination: Narrative and the symbolic boundaries between medicine and nursing. *Journal of Advanced Nursing, 25*(5), 1094–1100.

May, C. R., & Purkis, M. E. (1995). The configuration of nurse–patient relationships: A critical view. *Scholarly Inquiry for Nursing Practice, 9*(4), 283–295.

Meleis, A. I. (1997). *Theoretical nursing: Development and progress* (3rd ed.). Lippincott.

Meleis, A. I. (2007). *Theoretical nursing: Development and progress* (4th ed.). Lippincott Williams & Wilkins.

Nelson, S. (2000). *A genealogy of care of the sick: Nursing, holism and pious practice.* Nursing Praxis International.

Nelson, S. (2003). A history of small things. In J. Latimer (Ed.), *Advanced qualitative research for nursing* (pp. 211–230). Blackwell Science Ltd.

Paley, J. (2004). Gadow's romanticism: Science, poetry and embodiment in postmodern nursing. *Nursing Philosophy, 5*(2), 112–126.

Porter, S. (1998). *Social theory and nursing practice*. Macmillan Education UK.

Porter, S., & O'Halloran, P. (2009). The postmodernist war on evidence-based practice. *International Journal of Nursing Studies, 46*(5), 740–748.

Porter, S., & O'Halloran, P. (2010). Postmodernism and evidence-based practice: A reply to Holmes et al. *International Journal of Nursing Studies, 47*(4), 529–530.

Purkis, M. E. (1994). Entering the field: Intrusions of the social and its exclusion from studies of nursing practice. *International Journal of Nursing Studies, 31*(4), 315–336.

Purkis, M. E. (2013). Mary Ellen Purkis. In A. Forss, C. Ceci, & J. S. Drummond (Eds.), *Philosophy of nursing: 5 questions* (pp. 157–167). Automatic Press/VIP.

Purkis, M. E., & Bjornsdottir, K. (2006). Intelligent nursing: Accounting for knowledge as action in practice. *Nursing Philosophy, 7*(4), 247–256.

Reed, P. G., & Shearer, N. B. C. (2009). *Perspectives on nursing theory* (5th ed.). Wolters Kluwer/Lippincott Williams & Wilkins.

Risjord, M. (2010). *Nursing knowledge: Science, practice, and philosophy*. Wiley-Blackwell.

Rolfe, G. (2000). *Research, truth, and authority: Postmodern perspectives on nursing*. Macmillan Press.

Rudge, T., & Holmes, D. (Eds.). (2010). *Abjectly boundless: Bodies, boundaries and health work*. Ashgate.

Sandelowski, M. (1998). Looking to care or caring to look? Technology and the rise of spectacular nursing. *Holistic Nursing Practice, 12*(4), 1–11.

Sandelowski, M. (2002). Visible humans, vanishing bodies, and virtual nursing: Complications of life, presence, place, and identity. *Advances in Nursing Science, 24*(3), 58–70.

Sandelowski, M. (2003). Response to Dave Holmes and Cary Federman: Killing for the state: The darkest side of American nursing. *Nursing Inquiry, 10*(2), 139.

Seibold, C. (2000). Qualitative research from a feminist perspective in the postmodern era: Methodological, ethical and reflexive concerns. *Nursing Inquiry, 7*(3), 147–155.

Thorne, S. (2014). Nursing as social justice: A case for emancipatory disciplinary theorizing. In P. N. Kagan, M. C. Smith, & P. L. Chinn (Eds.), *Philosophies and practices of emancipatory nursing: Social justice as praxis* (pp. 79–92). Routledge.

Tschanz, C. (2005). To illustrate. In G. H. Doane & C. Varcoe (Eds.), *Family nursing as relational inquiry: Developing health-promoting practice* (p. 110). Lippincott Williams & Wilkins.

Traynor, M. (1997). Postmodern research: No grounding or privilege, just free-floating trouble making. *Nursing Inquiry, 4*(2), 99–107.

Traynor, M. (2003). Discourse analysis, ideology and professional practice. In J. Latimer (Ed.), *Advanced qualitative research for nursing* (pp. 137–154). Blackwell Science Ltd.

Traynor, M. (2006). Discourse analysis: Theoretical and historical overview and review of papers in the Journal of Advanced Nursing 1996–2004. *Journal of Advanced Nursing, 54*(1), 62–72.

Traynor, M. (2013). Discourse analysis. In C. T. Beck (Ed.), *The Routledge international handbook of qualitative nursing research* (pp. 282–294). Routledge.

Wied, S. (2006). The concept of interaction in theory and practice. In H. S. Kim & I. Kollak (Eds.), *Nursing theories: Conceptual and philosophical foundations* (2nd ed., pp. 54–70). Springer Publishing Company.

7 It's Not About Being Comfortable Bedfellows

Why Postmodern and Post-structural Literacy Matters in Nursing

A Review of the Book's Arguments

The first citation to Foucault's work appeared in the British journal, *Journal of Advanced Nursing* (Lees et al., 1987) closely followed by the first mention of post-structuralism in the American journal *Advances in Nursing Science* (ANS; Dzurec, 1989). In the 1990s, many articles in nursing journals[1] and selected textbooks (mostly outside the United States) referred to postmodernism and post-structuralism. These references ranged from detailed expositions of key postmodern and post-structural concepts such as discourse and power to brief parenthetical references to Foucault's critique of the clinical gaze. In 1994, the launch of *Nursing Inquiry* journal under the leadership of two Australian nurse scholars – founding editor Judith Parker and later Sioban Nelson – greatly encouraged Foucauldian (and other theoretical) nursing writings. Continental philosophical nursing scholarship including its postmodern/post-structural streams was also actively promoted in the latter half of the 1990s by Scottish nurse-philosopher John Drummond through International Philosophy of Nursing conferences. In the American context, throughout the 1990s, a small group of scholars mostly connected to the University of Washington nursing program, which I called the *enclave group*, advocated critical, feminist, and postmodern approaches to nursing scholarship – via their well-informed publications and conferences.

The turn of the century was marked by an increasing visibility of postmodern and post-structural nursing scholarship outside the United States through publication of several books, a launch of a new journal, and the formation of scholarly groups. Books on the topic of postmodern nursing research included those by Cheek (2000), Rolfe (2000), and Latimer (2003; selected chapters);[2] a historiography informed by Foucault's notion of *care of the self* (Nelson, 2000) summarized in the previous chapter; an edited collection theorizing the body in nursing (Lawler, 1997); and a textbook surveying social theory, including postmodern and Foucault's work, and their relevance to nursing practice (Porter, 1998; although the author revealed his critical position towards Foucault's ideas). In 2000, a new journal *Nursing Philosophy* was established with a broad philosophical mandate. This journal became the official publication of the International Philosophy of

DOI: 10.4324/9781003194439-7

Nursing Society (IPONS) launched in 2003 at the 7th International Philosophy of Nursing Conference held at the University of Stirling in Scotland. Another nurse scholars-led international group, *In Sickness and In Health*, was formed with a strong Foucauldian focus. Table A3 lists nursing books citing Foucault from the late 1980s to the end of 2015.

In the *American* theoretical nursing context, the turn-of-the-century years were also marked by two noticeable publications referring to postmodernism and post-structuralism. One was an anthology of philosophy of science in nursing (Polifroni & Welch, 1999) with a chapter on "Postmodernism and Nursing Science" comprised of articles by Jean Watson (1995), Pamela Reed (1995), and Laura Dzurec (1989). The other advance was a thematic issue of the *ANS* journal in 2003 devoted to critical and postmodern perspectives. The aforementioned non-American and American publications around the year 2000 underscore three features in American nursing literature. It was characterized by far fewer relevant publications; a tendency to amicably lodge postmodern/post-structural notions within the discussions of philosophy of science, philosophy of nursing science, and American nursing theory; and a marked ignorance of wider postmodern/post-structural nursing work (despite the latter's critical attention to American "unique nursing science/theory").

In the American nursing literature, postmodern and post-structural ideas were overwhelmingly embedded – explicitly or implicitly – in a specific disciplinary framework. This framework, what I call the *American nursing matrix*, was established in the discipline of nursing in the United States from roughly the 1960s onwards and solidified in the 1970s–1980s, when a consensus was formed about a particular conception of science (as unique, discipline-specific, comprised of incommensurable paradigms, with a few metaparadigm concepts guiding knowledge development) and a particular conception of theory (located at various levels of abstraction, comprised of concepts, the "building blocks" that can be "clarified" at the outset of the process of "theory construction"). Risjord (2010), an American philosopher of science who examined nursing metatheoretical literature, demonstrated that these conceptions of science and theory (permeating American nursing theory literature to this day) were rooted in mid-20th-century logical positivism and its later criticisms (e.g. by Kuhn), but that all these views have long been rejected by philosophers and superseded by subsequent ideas in the philosophy of science.

Risjord (2010) surfaced the unacknowledged and entrenched legacy of the logical positivist conception of science in American nursing theory. At the time that Risjord was publishing his critique of nursing's historical engagement with philosophy and theory construction, nurse theorists expressed a contradictory but consensual view that a positivist legacy manifests as the use of the scientific method and a reductionist view of human beings. Countering this stance, Risjord argued that logical positivism manifests quite differently: as the infiltration of a particular image of theory into the American (meta)theoretical nursing writings. Building on Risjord's argument, I discerned the following "formalized" images of theory common to American nursing science (Petrovskaya et al., 2019). Theory is aligned with a corresponding "paradigm" to "properly" guide research. Theory's intelligibility and credibility rely on the explicit delineation of "concepts," their "interrelations," and "assumptions." Theory in some cases needs the rhetorical crutch of the "double-helix structure" of theory/research to convince the audience of the theory's "inseparability" from research. Theory is explicitly announced and named in the paper title so that no mistake is made about the author's "theoretical orientation." Theory is fitted into "big cause" discourse (such as humanistic science or emancipatory practice) to guarantee theory's place in proper "nursing knowledge." Theory's "ethical currency" is made obvious through converting it into a "framework" to "guide practice." Bringing together insights of Risjord (2010) and Nelson (2000), two strong critics of American nursing theory, but occupying very different theoretical positions, I argued that theoretical writings/ theorizing of nursing practice that did not conform rhetorically or ideologically to these precepts risked remaining not only invisible but also unintelligible.

Throughout the chapters, I walked the reader through various permutations of the American nursing matrix: Fawcett's "structure of nursing knowledge"; *Nursing Science Quarterly's* unequivocal position that any "borrowed" theory should be connected to extant nursing models and theoretical frameworks in order to count as "nursing knowledge"; Reed's advocacy for theories generated from practice in such a way that "metanarratives" in the form of nursing's human science should provide the values guiding the process; and Chinn's model of knowledge development built upon Carper's "ways of knowing" that promoted integration among various elements of nursing knowledge from grand theories to practice theories and that incorporated critical, feminist, and postmodern/ post-structural nursing scholarship under the "emancipatory way of knowing." Throughout the chapters, I focused on how this intellectual matrix severely constrained the visibility and intelligibility of postmodern and post-structural insights in most American nursing literature. Postmodern and post-structural ideas were read highly selectively to strengthen anti-(medical)science rhetoric and to support humanistic and emancipatory agendas (vaguely and eclectically conceived, from a theoretical point a view) of knowledge generation. In other words, the concerns of many American publications deploying postmodern/post-structural ideas were limited to the discipline of nursing itself, its knowledge-generation activities, and philosophy of "unique nursing science." In contrast, the non-romantic understanding of nursing *practice* and the *critical* evaluation of the canon of American nursing science/theory – two contributions that postmodern and post-structural theory is so capable of (as I illustrated with the examples of the enclave group and non-American nursing scholarship) – fell outside of and were rendered unintelligible by the dominant disciplinary matrix in the United States. Indeed, those American nurse authors who applied postmodern and post-structural theories outside of "unique nursing science," for example, the enclave group, became visible on the "nursing knowledge" terrain mostly when their writings were connected to some larger metanarrative such as "emancipatory praxis" (e.g. in Kagan et al., 2014).

Within the American nursing matrix, writings framed by their authors as "nursing science and nursing theory" (e.g. Polifroni, 2010; Reed, 1995; Watson,1995,

1999), advocating epistemic diversity (e.g. Dzurec, 1989; Georges, 2003), or pursuing "emancipatory ways of knowing" (e.g. Chinn) produced either over-simplified or caricature representations of postmodernism, post-structuralism, and Foucault, as I have shown in Chapters 4 and 5. The enclave group, in their work, maintained distance from "unique nursing science" but were nevertheless involved in the discourse of nursing theory through their publications in *ANS* and some anthologies of "nursing knowledge" (Thompson, 2007, in Roy & Jones, 2007). These well-informed readings of Foucault and postmodern feminist lit-erature by the enclave nurses were likely unintelligible within the matrix – their meaning overdetermined by the "postmodern" work just listed. On the other hand, those rare American nurse scholars aptly doing the very postmodern work of contesting binary oppositions like Sandelowski (1999, 2002, Barnard & Sand-elowski, 2001), have not claimed the postmodern territory.

Noteworthy, the term *postmodernism* has been tainted in the United States and Europe in the late 1990s by what is referred to as the "Sokal affair" (Cusset, 2008, pp. 2–7; Rolfe, 2000, p. 45).[3] The echoes of the Sokal affair are heard in nursing in Glazer's (2001) and Garrett's (2018) criticisms of certain American nursing theory that somehow became associated with "postmodernism." (Indeed, some American publications like Koerner, 1996, associated nursing theories said to be informed by quantum physics with the "postmodern worldview.") What we are dealing with, then, is a jumble of misreadings and criticisms of postmodern and post-structural theory that might have kept some nurses from entering this tangled knot.

As far as I am aware, this book is the first systematic attempt to bring together the vast field of postmodern and post-structural nursing writings generated from the late 1980s through the first decade of 2000s. My specific focus was on compar-ing the application of postmodern, post-structural, and Foucault's ideas in Ameri-can nursing theory on the one hand and publications by the American enclave group and selected non-American authors on the other. Whereas I undertook a nearly comprehensive overview of American writings (Tables A1 and A2), I focused on a few pioneering and prominent non-American examples. This per-spective allowed me to create and sharpen the contrast between these two bod-ies of writings, while also noticing the heterogeneity within them. For example, within the non-American postmodern/post-structural field, I pointed out criti-cisms of Foucault's work by Porter (1994, 1996, 1997; Porter & O'Halloran, 2009, 2010). My intent in this book is to contribute to a better understanding of various practices of theorizing in the discipline of nursing.

Towards an Explanation of the Phenomenon of American Nursing Theory and Its Immunity to (Continental Philosophical) Criticisms

American nursing theory, as I have argued in this book, is a unique phenom-enon in the discipline, and there are several possible explanations for the way it arose and took hold of nursing theoretical discourse in the United States. As I speculate in the following, the circumstances of nursing's entry into the academy coupled with the distinctive "political consciousness" of the United States set the stage for American nursing theory to emerge. Further, American exceptionalism and capitalist ethos of the academy are two powerful forces in American life that may have had a role in the emergence of American nursing theory with both its insularism and acceptance of nursing theorists/theories as branded business models.

The Climate of Nursing's Entry Into the Academy

The growth of the academic discipline of nursing in the United States in the 1950s–1970s coincided with the waning but still influential role of the logical empiricist philosophy of science and Kuhn's criticisms of this view – ideas nurses relied upon to formulate a philosophy of nursing science (Risjord, 2010). In contrast, in Australia and the United Kingdom, other intellectual currents prevailed in the academy at large when nursing moved to higher education later in the 20th century.

That an *Australian* nurse was the first to *explicitly* introduce Foucault to the nursing audiences on the pages of the *Journal of Advanced Nursing* (Henderson, 1994) is not surprising considering the noticeable interest Australian nurse academics displayed towards German and French critical philosophy while also "trying on" American nursing theory. Australia and New Zealand were ahead of Canada and the United Kingdom in reforms of nursing education that resulted in a transfer of pre-licensure, or undergraduate, education to a tertiary, university sector. This process was uneven and lengthy, occurring in Australia mostly in the 1980s (Nelson, 2000, p. 20), in Canada roughly during the 1990s, and in the United Kingdom in the late 1990s and into the 21st century (Rolfe, 2000, p. xi). The creation of academic nursing programs inevitably led to the emergence of an interest in theory and research among new nursing faculty. Alongside this emergence, the discipline of nursing underwent professionalization, which required an edifice of abstract knowledge as evidenced in American nursing theory (see Chapter 3 for a reference to Abbott's work on this).

Australian nursing publications from the 1990s offer a glimpse into the diverse theoretical grounds of its authors. In fact, bibliographies reveal their authors' enviable familiarity with the debates in the American humanities and social sciences such as feminism/postmodernism debates (e.g. Heslop, 1997). As early as 1991, French philosophers were cited in an edited Australian textbook on professional issues in nursing (Gray & Pratt, 1991) and in a study of the *body* in nursing by a nurse sociologist Lawler (1991). But the most significant and lasting contribution to Foucauldian scholarship in our discipline occurred in 1994 – the launch of *Nursing Inquiry*, led by Australian nurses with the humanities background, J. Parker and Nelson. Thus, the academic nursing landscape in Australia differed markedly from that in the United States. As Gastaldo and D. Holmes (1999) speculate, "The limited influence of nursing models and theory in Australia [as compared with North America] has left room for nurses to explore more interdisciplinary theoretical perspectives, such as Foucault's" (p. 233). To summarize, curricular decisions and politics of nursing knowledge in different countries emerge as a powerful condition of possibility for kinds of theoretical knowledge deemed important for nursing students and encouraged by the discipline of nursing.

U.S. and Other Countries' Receptivity to Continental Philosophy

Various commentators, in nursing and beyond, pointed out historically produced differences in "political consciousness" (my phrase) among citizens of different countries. For example, German and British Marxism is said to be frowned upon in the United States, whereas Australia is described as a hotbed of critical theory. In a nursing context, Perron and Rudge (2016) observe that in the mid-20th century the development of nursing knowledge in the United States has been influenced by the (limiting) scientific model as well as a sociological perspective of structural functionalism. Extending feminist philosopher of science Harding's (2006) criticism of the rejection of ideas of Freud and Marx by American philosophy of science, Perron and Rudge observe that, similarly, in nursing "dangerous knowledge such as Freudian and Marxian thought was cast aside" (p. 47).[4]

American Exceptionalism

American exceptionalism – a well-known phenomenon – may partially explain parochial tendencies of American nurse theorists. One should be careful not to overstate the essentialist nature of this phenomenon; after all, literature also mentions British and other exceptionalisms. Yet, from the exceptionalist language peppered through Puritan John Winthrop's sermons in the 1600s to Obama's reshaping of America as imperfect yet exceptional (Fournier, 2016), there has long been a sense that America has a special destiny, and its people are unique (Madsen, 1998). A 2010 Gallup poll showed that 80 percent of Americans agreed with the statement, "The United States has a unique character because of its history and Constitution that sets it apart from other nations as the greatest in the world" (Jones, 2010). However, American exceptionalists need not love everything about America; they may fiercely criticize America's flaws, but those flaws are uniquely American and therefore exceptional.

American exceptionalist ideology has been contested in academia since the 1970s, with scholars pointing out the paradoxes inherent in the idea of exceptionalism (Gutfield, 2002) and others calling it a myth (Cheyfitz, 2009; Walter, 2011). Nonetheless, according to Cheyfitz, there continues to be support for American exceptionalism in the "corporate" university environment; protecting American exceptionalism protects the universities' profits.

American exceptionalism, then, might simply be part of the milieu of American life. It might be speculated that American scholars educated in elite universities especially prior to the 1970s were socialized into the ideology of American exceptionalism and perhaps carried these biases into their academic careers. Here, perhaps, we may find one root of American nursing theory's insular tendencies. However, this phenomenon is not universal – I have set apart the so-called enclave group of American nurse scholars who do not fit this pattern.

Capitalist Ethos of American Nursing Theory

The case of American nursing theory presents an unconventional application of "theory" not paralleled in how theory is used in the humanities, for example. While nurse scholars may run consulting agencies and develop branded curricular and care models, some nursing theories are commodified to the degree that it is unclear whether the notion of scholarly debate and criticism still bears on these products. In other words, why would a nurse theorist bother with criticisms of their work if rather than aiming to refine a theory as a tool to explain the world they are selling theory as a lifestyle? One of the most illustrative examples is Jean Watson's "caring theory."

The Watson Caring Science Institute website includes a notable e-commerce element. Although the institute is non-profit, a "Shop" button on the main menu takes the viewer to several purchasing options: a gift store selling merchandise with the Caring Science lotus logo, such as candles, tote bags, t-shirts, and mugs; two "libraries" showcasing books for sale by Watson and others; "educational" products such as a "reflective journal" and Jean's "Caritas meditation" CD; and downloadable products. Additionally, the website sells different levels of membership, from $35 to $150 a year and copyrighted training for leaders and executives.

Watson's non-profit organization's core is "Caring Science," "Unitary Caring Science," and "Theory of Human Caring," theories/ideas developed during her years as a doctoral student and then professor of nursing. As we would expect, information about her theories has a prominent place on the website (first item on main menu). However, scholarly theory seems a strange bedfellow to "lifestyle" products, such as the $15 seven-chakras gemstone bracelet, the $20 Pashmina shawl, or "lavender calm and body bliss" cream. Although non-profits often sell products to fundraise, the products sold on Watson's website seem to fit more with a capitalist model than a non-profit model because the link between the organization's mission (to advance the unitary philosophies, theories, and practices of "Caring Science") and the products often seems tenuous. It may be that Watson's philosophies and theories – a combination of New Age spiritual ideas – lend themselves to a wide array of products that suggest self-care, caring, heart, connection, and Eastern religions/philosophies. Further, the theory excerpts on the website look like a collection of aspirational claims that can be easily packaged as vision, mission, and philosophy statements about caring for organizations and nursing care delivery models.

In the world of social sciences and humanities, I am not aware of any parallels to Watson's commodification of theory. Academics frequently host their own personal or academic/professional websites where they may sell their books, and sometimes scholars serve as consultants to governments. For example, based on their analyses of social issues, Lyotard consulted the Quebec Government on matters of knowledge economy (Gratton, 2018) and Giddens advised the British prime minister (Britannica, 2022). Similarly, in the psychology world, psychometric tools developed by psychologists are sold on their personal websites. However, there is, to my knowledge, no equivalent to Watson's combination of theory and e-commerce for revenue generation. Here, then, is another difference between American nursing theory and other forms of theorizing in nursing: theory as a product in a capitalist context, to which the notions of "theory refinement" or "scholarly debate" no longer apply.

Significance of This Book for Nursing Research, Education, and Clinical Practice

The relationship between the argument in this book and clinical nursing practice is mediated by the process of education of nurses. The relevance of this book's argument lies in the ideational realm – in how nurses think about and understand their role, practice, nursing knowledge, and the profession. This realm, consequential for nurses' conduct, is part and parcel of nursing education. I discuss the significance of my research for education *and* practice in this section that concludes the book.

Representations of Nursing Practice in Theoretical Accounts: Same Goal Different Means?

It is quite uncontroversial to say that regardless of a specific perspective, different theoretical formulations of "nursing" pursue a similar goal – to help bring about better quality, humane nursing practice. These theoretical pronouncements, however, differ in how they hope to actualize this ideal. And this difference in means is not inconsequential – it generates effects for how nurses are socialized (textually, ideologically) into the world of nursing, how they are guided to describe their work to themselves and others, and what they take as legitimate professional concerns as opposed to interfering "white noise."

The ultimate nursing orientation understood and conveyed by disciplinary theoretical discourses (as diverse as American nursing theory, nursing philosophy of analytical leanings, or continental philosophy of nursing) – is that nursing practice at its best cannot be reduced to either a biomedical focus or economically driven technical efficiency. Nursing "caring" theorists, "unitary-transformative" theorists, "holistic" theorists, nurse phenomenologists, nurses drawing on ancient Greek philosophers, those influenced by critical theory, or postmodern/post-structural and other post-humanist theory – with all their legitimate theoretical (and hence practical-ideological) disagreements – share this orientation.

Historically, in the American context, much nursing theorizing arose from an anxiety around shifting nurses' roles and a desire to arm nurses with an ideological perspective that would enable them to stand the patient-centred ground amidst the countering priorities of profit-driven health care. (This concern arguably provides a strong current impetus for teaching nursing theory.) For instance, this focus on the *person* (persons' meanings of their experiences as lived) as the highest priority of nursing practice seems to ground Mitchell and Cody's (1992) insistence on the "unitary" nature of human beings opposed to "physical and psychological subsystems" reductionism. To these scholars, this position is uncompromising: Nurses either hold a unitary view (or a holistic view, in other theorists' terminology) as the highest value of professional nursing or subscribe to biomedical reductionism. The belief is that nurses' values, such as the holistic ideal, enable them to withstand the corrupting demands of the workplace: "Nurses cannot switch their very beliefs according to the nature of the practice situation" (Mitchell & Cody, 1992, p. 57). However, Risjord (2010, p. 151) retorts that, contrary to such a tenacious view, he can freely reconcile treating his daughter as a whole autonomous person while washing her scraped knee with an antimicrobial soap, as biomedical knowledge instructs. Risjord is right, and yet there might be something else at stake behind Mitchell and Cody's insistence, which many nurses would recognize. I refer to the awareness of how easy it is to give up one's (i.e. nurse's ideal and perhaps idealistic) ground under the pressures of the system. Examples of acquiescence common in a hospital ward are well known, for instance, from insights offered by institutional ethnography studies: "nursing the chart" rather than nursing the patient (MacKinnon & McIntyre, 2006) or unquestioningly accepting the priority of "moving" patients through the system faster (Rankin & M. Campbell, 2006). A question arises: Does the canon of American nursing theory offer theoretical tools to help nurses understand, "get through," and question the current realities of nursing practice? Is an "ideal vision" of nursing (e.g. Watson, Chinn) capable of analysis, for example, of *how* nurses get "enrolled" into managerial technologies of efficiency and effectiveness (Rudge, 2013)?

An intractable issue with the "ideal vision" offered by some well-known nurse theorizing is that it presents an ahistorical and acontextual image of nursing: a view of nursing practice as an insular, caring, patient-centred encounter where a benevolent nurse empowers clients; a view of holistic nursing theory as an evolutionary pinnacle; and a view of "nursing inquiry" as hostile towards biomedical "positivism" or at least comprising a unique "knowledge paradigm" coexisting but incommensurate with other "paradigms." This fixed image lies at the "foundation" of the nursing's "unique" disciplinary knowledge.

It appears that nursing writings and genres adhering to one or another version of this intellectual "foundation" (and that operate with particular formal terminology, that is, grand theory, middle-range theory, practice-level theory, borrowed theory, metaparadigm, paradigms, or models of knowledge development based on "patterns of knowing") have been granted "nursing knowledge" status, making other conceptions of theory as well as practices of theorizing unintelligible forms of nursing knowledge (Petrovskaya et al., 2019). As I have argued, the domain of "unique nursing science" is highly problematic on two grounds – as a conception of science rooted in the outdated logical positivist view (Risjord, 2010) as well as a professional ideology of holism presenting the holistic nurse as a preferred ethical persona (Nelson, 2000) and a holistic nurse–patient relationship as an unproblematic and power-free access to "the real" person who is to be known (May, 1992a, 1992b, 1995a, 1995b).

My study brings into the spotlight another kind of theorizing in our discipline. The radical potential of postmodern and post-structural French theory – its conceptual toolbox – has been embraced by non-American and some American nurses (whose work published in the 1990s and early 2000s I examined) to think through questions of nursing practice, nursing research, and nursing history. Their theorizing did not seek to transcend the "realities" of nursing practice in search for some idealized "disciplinary core," but rather paid close attention to the socio-political context of everyday practice.

The theoretical accounts of nursing practice that I singled out as particularly interesting examples of scholarship informed by postmodern/post-structural ideas attempt to reach nursing students not through indoctrination or a metaphysical conversion – technologies to enhance modern subjectivity (Nelson, 1995) – but through alternative mechanisms. Nelson (1995) describes this alternative approach:

> Nursing is often conceptualized as an art and a science, a dynamic balance between aesthetic, humanist and scientific practices. A different approach is to start from the view that nursing is a set of practices or technologies that do not stand in need of unification at a higher level in the form of an all-encompassing belief system or doctrine. From this vantage point the dichotomy between science and spirituality is unhelpful if the object is to better describe the elements of practice in their own terms, rather than in terms of the formation of the subject. Practices of specific derivation are assembled in a number of contexts, the hybrid manner in which this occurs is various and historically contingent, rather than deriving from or depending on a single general explanation or unifying principle. These assemblages of actions form the cultural complex that now constitutes nursing. . . . This allows for a better appreciation of the complexities of modern nursing.
>
> (p. 41)

These alternative mechanisms present nursing practices as hybrid activities (involving human actors and technology; "human" and technical skills) that do not require unifying metaphysical narratives; that teach nurses to think, examine assumptions, and raise questions (broadly the task of philosophy); and that invite nurses to understand the realities of nursing practice as socially accomplished processes involving many actors, technology, professional cultures, organizational context, and wider socio-economic factors. These theoretical attempts defamiliarize commonsense perceptions of practice and ask why it is so difficult to carve out time for an "ideal caring moment," how "getting to know the patient" is not always a benevolent move, how texts (e.g. guidelines, health records) direct nurses' attention, and who is entitled to speak on matters of health and illness. But importantly, the answers offered in these theoretical accounts stay away from romantic or moralistic terms and from making the "medical model" a villain. I believe it is important for nursing students to be introduced to this body of theoretical work in the discipline of nursing.

The Focus on Critical Theoretical Nursing Discourse

One goal of my book was to bring into view robust criticisms generated in nursing and challenging influential theoretical ideas. From the late 1980s and into the 2000s, American nursing theory turned a blind eye not only towards continental and social theory as useful for nursing practice and scholarship but also towards any critiques directed at nursing theory – critiques from analytic philosophical perspectives (Edwards, 1999, 2001; Kikuchi, 2003, 2008; selected chapters in Kim & Kollak, 2006; Paley, 2001, 2002, 2006; Risjord, 2010) or continental philosophical and social-theoretical perspectives (Davina Allen, 2014; Drevdahl, 1999; Drummond, 2013; selected chapters in Kim & Kollak, 2006; Mulholland, 1995; Nelson, 2000; Purkis, 1994, 1997). American nursing theory textbooks, such as the famous multi-edition volume *Nursing Theorists and Their Work* (Alligood, 2014; Alligood & Tomey, 2010; Tomey & Alligood, 2006), were an important source that initiated nursing students into the world of theory. However, the image of theory held out to nursing students is serenely uncritical and thus lacks scholarly quality (Paley, 2006). I drew upon several books that critically examine established disciplinary ideas – books by Davina Allen (2015), Forss et al. (2013), Kim and Kollak (2006), Latimer (2003), Nelson (2000), Risjord (2010), Sandelowski (2000a), and Thompson et al. (1992). It appears to me that these sources do not enjoy the status they deserve – as an important component of nursing curricula. Yet these texts can invigorate and add quality to theoretical discussions in the nursing classroom.

The notion of an American nursing (theoretical, disciplinary) matrix of (un) intelligibility has been threaded throughout my argument. We can think about this matrix not only as certain mental habits of thinkers but as practices that produced textual effects – codified ways to generate knowledge and write about nursing. I argued that not only did this matrix passively exclude certain philosophical ideas, thus making them marginal and invisible, it also actively produced unintelligibility via an additive, cumulative mode of inclusion. (The additive mode refers to a simple accumulation of new ideas and "patterns of knowing" in a spirit of "multiple-ism" without a revision of the established beliefs.) Only that which was both included into the matrix (or its versions) and made alike with its other elements was legitimated and gained intelligibility as "nursing knowledge" in American nursing *theoretical* journals and textbooks on nursing theory. It seems that as long as the American intellectual matrix (the structure of nursing knowledge à la Fawcett, the models of theory development à la L. O. Walker and Avant, the integrative conceptions of nursing science) dominates the discipline's theoretical imagination, contemporary continental philosophy/social theory will remain in a lose–lose situation in American theoretical discourse (Petrovskaya et al., 2019).

Importantly, a distinctive critical edge of post-structuralism relates to its theoretical anti-humanism (Soper, 1986). Granted, the word *anti-humanism* sounds off-putting especially when one does not understand it. Perhaps due to this, some nursing literature exhibits a curious inability to fully explore the potential and implications of Foucault's post-structuralism. Some nurse authors who offered critical readings of nursing issues (e.g. Foucault-based analyses) were nevertheless compelled – often unwittingly, perhaps following disciplinary conventions – to produce a "happy ending." A case in point is a critique of clinical supervision in the United Kingdom by Freshwater et al. (2015). Clinical supervision is a quality improvement mechanism requiring nurses to reflect on clinical situations through conversations with an experienced colleague. Freshwater et al. (2015) fittingly applied Foucault's notions of surveillance and confession to reveal the Panopticon nature of clinical supervision. Then, however, the authors turned to contrasting two kinds of nurse: the "artificial person" (p. 8), who resists those "reflexive" opportunities likely because she has internalized the institutional climate of suspicion, and a preferred kind, the "autonomous individual" (p. 8). The latter nurse is also immersed in this institutional climate, but readily engages in conversations with a clinical supervisor (who happens to be a psychotherapist trained in humanistic psychology) to critically evaluate how those institutional discourses have colonized nurse's authentic caring self.

Indeed, Foucault's work implicates nursing in the "sciences of Man," in the practices of disciplinary societies, and in the exercise of governmentality (that flows from nurses to patients and from nurse supervisors to rank-and-file nurses) – all techniques of power in 20th century Western societies. Thus, some writings based on Foucault's ideas, such as by Freshwater and colleagues, appear to convey nurse authors' discomfort, perhaps unavoidable, considering the aforementioned claim. This article and other similar ones, despite the authors' apparent alignment with Foucault, reflect the stronghold of humanistic ideals in the authors' conceptions of the "helping professions" or at least an obligation to optimistically posit a "more critical and authentic nurse." Echoing these observations, Traynor (2006) commented on a tendency of nurse researchers engaged in discourse-analytic studies to read Foucault's work in a humanistic vein.

In contrast to these selected *nursing* works, some social scientists and humanities scholars (or nurses with background in these fields) studying nursing practice (e.g. Davina Allen, Latimer, Nelson, Paley, Risjord, Traynor) were able to hold a more theoretically robust and less flattering mirror to the nursing discipline and the profession. I perceive this as the strength of these authors' analyses.

There might be another reason to attempt to understand theoretical anti-humanism: as a precursor for nurse scholars' ability to engage with other perspectives not aligned with the philosophical assumptions of Western humanism. Instead of misinterpreting theoretical anti-humanism as a call to somehow abandon humane nursing care, it has been applied in the best Foucauldian nursing analyses to a different effect as I have shown throughout the chapters. Foucault's theoretical anti-humanism alongside other related perspectives invited a shift in scholars' attention away from nurses' attitudes and intentions to the events and materialities of nursing practice accomplished in organizational contexts. Nurse scholars' ability to appreciate a post-structural decentring of the human subject indicates their ability to rigorously engage with other contemporary strands of social, cultural, and political theory. For example, actor network theory (Latour, 2005) and its "post" varieties (Mol, 2021), animal studies (Lennard & Wolfe, 2017) and writings on "companion species" by Donna Haraway (Gane, 2006), posthumanism (Braidotti, 2013; Hayles, 1999), new materialism (Barad, 2003; see Aranda, 2017, for a nursing example), versions of environmentalism, and Indigenous perspectives do not afford humans an omnipotent place at the top of the hierarchy of life. While nurse theorists might be interested in these perspectives (to endorse or criticize them), I doubt the intelligibility of these theories within the American nursing theoretical matrix.

Awareness of Limitations of Curricular Categories

The commonsense curricular divisions such as "(American) nursing theory" or "qualitative research" along which nursing courses are designed may leave out a sizable and important body of writings, specifically continental nursing philosophy and nursing history. The main purpose of my study was to understand how the intellectual landscape of the nursing discipline has shaped, and continues to shape, a recognition and reception of continental philosophical scholarship, specifically nursing writings informed by postmodern and post-structural theory. Within this scholarly landscape, I attended to the distinctive (but sometimes overlapping) discourses of nursing science, qualitative research, and nursing philosophy. I argued that certain assumptions and discursive constructs mobilized within American conceptions of theory leave little room for continentally informed nursing scholarship, particularly those ideas sceptical of humanistic and emancipatory agendas. Continental theorizing in nursing produced numerous clinically significant and textually interesting analyses. They, however, may not fit the frame of nursing science and nursing theory, a genre of qualitative research, or certain forms of nursing philosophy. This creates problems for all parties: Nursing continental theorizing of a post-humanist kind remains at the margins, which prevents a robust critical engagement with this branch of scholarship (including the necessity to address the ongoing issue of its theoretical rigour or accurate reading of philosophy). On the other hand, established "nursing knowledge" remains largely immune to continental philosophical criticisms. I draw attention to the intellectual blinders imposed by curricular rubrics so that a less rigid categorization of scholarship can be embraced, and the writings hitherto "unintelligible" can find their way into course syllabi.

A detailed analysis of nursing literature informed by postmodern/post-structural theory during the first two decades of this field, particularly of its American nursing theory stream as contrasted with the enclave group's and selected non-American works, enables nurse readers to appreciate this field of nursing scholarship and to understand it in the context of other disciplinary ideas. The importance of this book lies in its potential to enhance nurse readers' and researchers' literacy when dealing with nursing and social scientific studies informed by postmodern and post-structural theory.

Notes

1 Thinking of the entire body of nursing scholarship during the decade of the 1990s, very few papers – in the context of the whole – take up postmodern/post-structural ideas. In my estimation, based on CINAHL searches supplemented by hand searches, before the year 2000, slightly over 100 journal articles mentioned Foucault: the overwhelming majority in the *Journal of Advanced Nursing* and *Nursing Inquiry* and a handful in *Advances in Nursing Science*. Two journals that were not easily retrievable via electronic searches, *International Journal of Nursing Studies* (*IJNS*) and *Scholarly Inquiry for Nursing Practice* (*SINP*), are worth mentioning. Many interesting articles cited throughout the book, including those citing Foucault, come from these journals. Established in 1963, *IJNS* has been geared to the international nursing audience, focused on research, and not engrossed in the American nursing theory movement. In the 1990s, *IJNS* articles by Purkis (1994), Cheek and Rudge (1994), and Kermode and Brown (1996) cited Foucault or referred to postmodernism. After 2010, *IJNS* appears to have shifted away from theoretical and philosophical papers towards publishing systematic reviews, randomized trials, and metasyntheses.

In turn, *SINP* was established in 1987 and renamed in 2002 as *Research and Theory for Nursing Practice*. An interesting and unique feature of this journal was that responses accompanied most articles. It appears that in the 1990s, *SINP* was a meeting place between British and American nursing perspectives as well as between American perspectives. Examples of the former include May and Purkis (1995) vis-à-vis Lowenberg (1995) on the nurse–patient relationship; Bjornsdottir (1998) vis-à-vis Liaschenko (1998) on language and power in nursing practice; and Paley (2000) vis-à-vis Sandelowski (2000b) on paradigms in qualitative research. Examples of the latter include Liaschenko (1997) vis-à-vis Chinn (1997) on the nature of feminist theorizing and Drevdahl (1998) vis-à-vis Thompson (1998) on the notion of "community."

2 Table A3 in the Appendix provides additional detail on the following books: Julianne Cheek's (2000) monograph *Postmodern and Poststructural Approaches to Nursing Research*; Gary Rolfe's (2000) anthology with a substantial author's introduction, *Research, Truth, and Authority: Postmodern Perspectives on Nursing*; and Joanna Latimer's (2003) edited anthology *Advanced Qualitative Research for Nursing*. Collectively, these texts illustrate a wide range of methodological concerns prompted by the continental movements of postmodernism and post-structuralism among social scientists and nurse researchers outside the United States. These concerns include attention to the notions of text, representation, selves, the role of the author/researcher, the nature of writing, discourse, and the constitutive role of language – concerns rarely raised by American nurse researchers.

Cheek (2000) and Rolfe (2000) undertake some of the earliest book-format expositions and summaries of key ideas of selected French philosophers for nursing audiences. Cheek's book is a guide on how to write a qualitative research proposal and how to systematically collect data for a study of media discourses. In turn, Rolfe's contribution to postmodern nursing scholarship, in this book and elsewhere, lies in his ability to convey the *pleasure of text* (à la Barthes and Derrida) and in his persistence in demonstrating the relevance of French literary theory for nursing. Part of Rolfe's book is organized as an anthology of five articles from nursing journals to illustrate diverse postmodern perspectives on nursing research. Rolfe skilfully teases out the points of agreement and disagreement among his own and others' viewpoints. For instance, he problematizes attempts to uncritically assimilate Foucault with a feminist emancipatory agenda (p. 155) and, in another case, questions the necessity to position postmodernism as a "new science" (pp. 131–132).

However, Cheek's (2000) but especially Rolfe's (2000) respective arguments rely on the construction of a rather dramatic contrast between two entities: modernist science and postmodern research. These authors tend to present postmodern and post-structural theories as lending themselves to the unique research approaches positioned as anti-(modernist) science. Their writings presuppose the quantitative/qualitative binary; however, Cheek explicitly advocates for discourse analysis as a qualitative methodology, whereas Rolfe attempts to extricate postmodern nursing research from any *science*, quantitative or qualitative.

Latimer's (2003) anthology presents some well-informed applications of postmodern and post-structural theory in the context of empirical (ethnographic, discourse-analytic, and historical) studies of nursing practice. These applications provide a stark contrast to both hardly existent American postmodern/post-structural nursing research and the qualitative-paradigmatic direction of non-American postmodern/post-structural methodological nursing literature discussed before (e.g. Cheek, 2000; Rolfe, 2000).

Some interesting and consequential features of methodological reflections in Latimer's (2003) book are scepticism towards the "psychologized subject"; avoidance of binary oppositions; a confident practice of interpretation; the "inseparability" of theory, research, and practice; and encouragement of certain stylistic features of research reports.

3　The Sokal Affair involved academic deception for the ostensible purpose of showing the negative influence of postmodern philosophy. In 1996, physics professor Alan Sokal submitted a hoax article to *Social Text*, a postmodern cultural studies journal. The article criticized the natural sciences for upholding a realist view of the world. Intentionally written in a nearly incomprehensible style, the article was peppered with phrases fashionable at the time in some cultural studies claiming French-theoretical postmodern influences. After the article was published, Sokal claimed that his goal was to show how humanities scholars and journals, negatively influenced by postmodern philosophy, were ready to buy into bogus criticisms of science without understanding it ("Sokal affair," 2022).

4　According to Perron and Rudge (2016), emancipatory and feminist ideas were latecomers to nursing. Three nursing works, all originating in the United States, are cited by Perron and Rudge as examples of the latter – David Allen (1985), an early publication by Annette Street, and Kagan et al. (2014). I certainly support Perron and Rudge's observation about kinds of theory unintelligible in the U.S. nursing theoretical scholarship (e.g. Freudian and Marxist). The forms of critical knowledge "external to nursing" were "subjugated" in our discipline (Perron & Rudge, 2016, p. 54). However, my research complicates this somewhat simplistic contrast between American "early/uncritical/scientific scholarship" and the "recent/emancipatory/radical" works generated in the American context. Specifically, within nursing's "emancipatory paradigm" (Chinn & Kramer, 2015), some kinds of theoretical analyses run the risk of being ignored. Partly, this might be an inevitable process – each knowledge creates its ignorance(s). But here we deal with another issue, which bypassed some streams of the non-American post-structural work (as my examples in Chapter 6 demonstrate). The issue lies not (only) with the "ideological conservatism" of the "traditional" nurse scientists in the sense of a conscious decision to censor specific theory as Perron and Rudge imply in relation to Freud and Marx – but with an inability to "notice" and to read theory as "intelligible" within the intellectual matrix of American "nursing science" (including its "emancipatory pattern" actively promoted in *Advances in Nursing Science*) composed of language of "paradigms," "theoretical frameworks," and "levels of theory."

References

Allen, D. G. (1985). Nursing research and social control: Alternate models of science that emphasize understanding and emancipation. *Image: The Journal of Nursing Scholarship*, *17*(2), 58–64.

Allen, D. G. (2014). Re-conceptualising holism in the contemporary nursing mandate: From individual to organisational relationships. *Social Science & Medicine*, *119*, 131–138.

Allen, D. G. (2015). *The invisible work of nurses: Hospitals, organisation and healthcare*. Routledge.

Alligood, M. R. (Ed.). (2014). *Nursing theorists and their work* (8th ed.). Mosby Elsevier.

Alligood, M. R., & Tomey, A. M. (Eds.). (2010). *Nursing theorists and their work* (7th ed.). Mosby Elsevier.

Aranda, K. (2017). Feminism and nursing: An un/easy alliance of silences and absences. In M. Lipscomb (Ed.), *Social theory and nursing* (pp. 144–158). Routledge.

Barad, K. (2003). Posthumanist performativity: Toward an understanding of how matter comes to matter. *Signs*, *28*(3), 801–831.

Barnard, A., & Sandelowski, M. (2001). Technology and humane nursing care: (Ir)reconcilable or invented difference. *Journal of Advanced Nursing*, *34*(3), 367–375.

Bjornsdottir, K. (1998). Language, ideology, and nursing practice. *Scholarly Inquiry for Nursing Practice*, *12*(4), 347–362.

Braidotti, R. (2013). *The posthuman*. Polity Press.

Britannica, T. Editors of Encyclopaedia. (2022, January 14). *Anthony Giddens. Encyclopedia Britannica*. www.britannica.com/biography/Anthony-Giddens

Cheek, J. (2000). *Postmodern and poststructural approaches to nursing research*. SAGE.

Cheek, J., & Rudge, T. (1994). The panopticon re-visited: An exploration of the social and political dimensions of contemporary health care and nursing practice. *International Journal of Nursing Studies*, *31*(6), 583–591.

Cheyfitz, E. (2009). The corporate university, academic freedom, and American exceptionalism. *South Atlantic Quarterly*, *108*(4), 701–722.

Chinn, P. L. (1997). Response to "Ethics and the geography of the nurse–patient relationship." *Scholarly Inquiry for Nursing Practice*, *11*(1), 61–63.

Chinn, P. L., & Kramer, M. K. (2015). *Knowledge development in nursing: Theory and process* (9th ed.). Elsevier Health Sciences.

Cusset, F. (2008). *French theory: How Foucault, Derrida, Deleuze, & Co. transformed the intellectual life of the United States* (J. Fort, Trans.). University of Minnesota Press.

Drevdahl, D. (1998). Diamond necklaces: Perspectives on power and the language of "community." *Scholarly Inquiry for Nursing Practice*, *12*(4), 303–317.

Drevdahl, D. (1999). Sailing beyond: Nursing theory and the person. *Advances in Nursing Science*, *21*(4), 1–13.

Drummond, J. S. (2013). John S. Drummond. In A. Forss, C. Ceci, & J. S. Drummond (Eds.), *Philosophy of nursing: 5 questions* (pp. 45–54). Automatic Press/VIP.

Dzurec, L. (1989). The necessity for and evolution of multiple paradigms for nursing research: A poststructuralist perspective. *Advances in Nursing Science*, *11*(4), 69–77.

Edwards, S. D. (1999). The idea of nursing science. *Journal of Advanced Nursing*, *29*(3), 563–569.

Edwards, S. D. (2001). *Philosophy of nursing: An introduction*. Palgrave Macmillan.

Forss, A., Ceci, C., & Drummond, J. S. (Eds.). (2013). *Philosophy of nursing: 5 questions*. Automatic Press/VIP.

Fournier, R. (2016, July 28). Obama's new American exceptionalism. *The Atlantic*. www.theatlantic.com/politics/archive/2016/07/obamas-new-american-exceptionalism/493415

Freshwater, D., Fisher, P., & Walsh, E. (2015). Revisiting the panopticon: Professional regulation, surveillance and sousveillance. *Nursing Inquiry*, *22*(1), 3–12.

Gane, N. (2006). When we have never been human, what is to be done? Interview with Donna Haraway. *Theory, Culture & Society*, *23*(7–8), 135–158. https://dx.doi.org/10.1177/0263276406069228

Garrett, B. (2018). *Empirical nursing: The art of evidence-based care*. Emerald Publishing Limited.

Gastaldo, D., & Holmes, D. (1999). Foucault and nursing: A history of the present. *Nursing Inquiry*, 6(4), 231–240.

Georges, J. (2003). An emerging discourse: Toward epistemic diversity in nursing. *Advances in Nursing Science*, 26(1), 44–52.

Glazer, S. (2001). Therapeutic touch and postmodernism in nursing. *Nursing Philosophy*, 2(3), 196–212.

Gratton, P. (2018). Jean François Lyotard. In E. N. Zalta (Ed.), *The Stanford encyclopedia of philosophy*. https://plato.stanford.edu/archives/win2018/entries/lyotard/

Gray, G., & Pratt, R. (Eds.). (1991). *Towards a discipline of nursing*. Churchill Livingstone.

Gutfield, A. (2002). *American exceptionalism: The effects of plenty on the American experience*. Sussex Academic Press.

Harding, S. (2006). Two influential theories of ignorance and philosophy's interests in ignoring them. *Hypatia*, 21(3), 20–36.

Hayles, K. N. (1999). *How we became posthuman: Virtual bodies in cybernetics, literature, and informatics*. University of Chicago Press.

Henderson, A. (1994). Power and knowledge in nursing practice: The contribution of Foucault. *Journal of Advanced Nursing*, 20(5), 935–939.

Heslop, L. (1997). The (im)possibilities of poststructuralist and critical social nursing inquiry. *Nursing Inquiry*, 4(1), 48–56.

Jones, J. M. (2010, December 22). Americans see U.S. as exceptional; 37% doubt Obama does. *Gallop Poll Report*. https://news.gallup.com/poll/145358/americans-exceptional-doubt-obama.aspx

Kagan, P. N., Smith, M. C., & Chinn, P. L. (Eds.). (2014). *Philosophies and practices of emancipatory nursing: Social justice as praxis*. Routledge.

Kermode, S., & Brown, C. (1996). The postmodernist hoax and its effects on nursing. *International Journal of Nursing Studies*, 33(4), 375–384.

Kikuchi, J. F. (2003). Nursing knowledge and the problem of worldviews. *Research and Theory for Nursing Practice*, 17(1), 7–17.

Kikuchi, J. F. (2008). Polemics, taste, and truth in nursing discourse. *Nursing Philosophy*, 9(4), 273–276.

Kim, H. S., & Kollak, I. (Eds.). (2006). *Nursing theories: Conceptual and philosophical foundations* (2nd ed.). Springer Publishing Company.

Koerner, J. G. (1996). Imagining the future for nursing administration and systems research. *Nursing Administration Quarterly*, 20(4), 1–11.

Latimer, J. (2003). *Advanced qualitative research for nursing*. Blackwell Science Ltd.

Latour, B. (2005). *Reassembling the social: An introduction to actor-network-theory*. Oxford University Press.

Lawler, J. (1991). *Behind the screens: Nursing, somology and the problem of the body*. Churchill Livingstone.

Lawler J. (Ed.). (1997). *The body in nursing: A collection of views*. W. B. Saunders Company.

Lees, G., Richman, J., Salauroo, M., & Warden, S. (1987). Quality assurance: Is it professional insurance? *Journal of Advanced Nursing*, 12(6), 719–727.

Lennard, N., & Wolfe, C. (2017, January 9). Is humanism really humane? *The New York Times*. www.nytimes.com/2017/01/09/opinion/is-humanism-really-humane.html

Liaschenko, J. (1997). Ethics and the geography of the nurse–patient relationship: Spatial vulnerabilities and gendered space. *Scholarly Inquiry for Nursing Practice*, 11(1), 45–59.

Liaschenko, J. (1998). Response to "Language, ideology, and nursing practice." *Scholarly Inquiry for Nursing Practice*, 12(4), 363–366.

Lowenberg, J. S. (1995). Response to "The configuration of nurse–patient relationships: A critical view." *Scholarly Inquiry for Nursing Practice, 9*(4), 297–301.

MacKinnon, K., & McIntyre, M. (2006). From Braxton Hicks to preterm labour: The constitution of risk in pregnancy. *Canadian Journal of Nursing Research, 38*(2), 56–72.

Madsen, D. L. (1998). *American exceptionalism*. University Press of Mississippi.

May, C. R. (1992a). Individual care – power and subjectivity in therapeutic relationships. *Sociology, 26*(4), 589–602.

May, C. R. (1992b). Nursing work, nurses' knowledge, and the subjectification of the patient. *Sociology of Health and Illness, 14*(4), 472–487.

May, C. R. (1995a). "To call it work somehow demeans it": The social construction of talk in the care of terminally ill patients. *Journal of Advanced Nursing, 22*(3), 556–561.

May, C. R. (1995b). Patient autonomy and the politics of professional relationships. *Journal of Advanced Nursing, 21*(1), 83–87.

May, C. R., & Purkis, M. E. (1995). The configuration of nurse–patient relationships: A critical view. *Scholarly Inquiry for Nursing Practice, 9*(4), 283–295.

Mitchell, G. J., & Cody, W. K. (1992). Nursing knowledge and human science: Ontological and epistemological considerations. *Nursing Science Quarterly, 5*, 54–61.

Mol, A. (2021). *Eating in theory*. Duke University Press.

Mulholland, J. (1995). Nursing, humanism and transcultural theory: The "bracketing-out" of reality. *Journal of Advanced Nursing, 22*(3), 442–449.

Nelson, S. (1995). Humanism in nursing: The emergence of the light. *Nursing Inquiry, 2*(1), 36–43.

Nelson, S. (2000). *A genealogy of care of the sick: Nursing, holism and pious practice*. Nursing Praxis International.

Paley, J. (2000). Paradigms and presuppositions: The difference between qualitative and quantitative research. *Scholarly Inquiry for Nursing Practice, 14*(2), 143–155.

Paley, J. (2001). An archaeology of caring knowledge. *Journal of Advanced Nursing, 36*(2), 188–198.

Paley, J. (2002). Caring as a slave morality: Nietzschean themes in nursing. *Journal of Advanced Nursing, 40*(1), 25–35.

Paley, J. (2006). Book review: Nursing theorists and their work. *Nursing Philosophy, 7*(4), 275–280.

Perron, A., & Rudge, T. (2016). *On the politics of ignorance in nursing and healthcare: Knowing ignorance*. Routledge.

Petrovskaya, O., Purkis, M. E., & Bjornsdottir, K. (2019). Revisiting "intelligent nursing": Olga Petrovskaya in conversation with Mary Ellen Purkis and Kristin Bjornsdottir. *Nursing Philosophy, 20*(3), e12259.

Polifroni, E. C. (2010). Power, right, and truth: Foucault's triangle as a model for clinical power. *Nursing Science Quarterly, 23*(1), 8–12.

Polifroni, E. C., & Welch, M. (Eds.). (1999). *Perspectives on philosophy of science in nursing: An historical and contemporary anthology*. Lippincott Williams & Wilkins.

Porter, S. (1994). New nursing: The road to freedom? *Journal of Advanced Nursing, 20*(2), 269–274.

Porter, S. (1996). Contra-Foucault: Soldiers, nurses and power. *Sociology, 30*(1), 59–78.

Porter, S. (1997). The patient and power: Sociological perspectives on the consequences of holistic care. *Health & Social Care in the Community, 5*(1), 17–20.

Porter, S. (1998). *Social theory and nursing practice*. Macmillan Education UK.

Porter, S., & O'Halloran, P. (2009). The postmodernist war on evidence-based practice. *International Journal of Nursing Studies, 46*(5), 740–748.

Porter, S., & O'Halloran, P. (2010). Postmodernism and evidence-based practice: A reply to Holmes et al. *International Journal of Nursing Studies, 47*(4), 529–530.

Purkis, M. E. (1994). Entering the field: Intrusions of the social and its exclusion from studies of nursing practice. *International Journal of Nursing Studies, 31*(4), 315–336.

Purkis, M. E. (1997). The "social determinants" of practice? A critical analysis of the discourse of health promotion. *The Canadian Journal of Nursing Research, 29*(1), 47–62.

Rankin, J. M., & Campbell, M. L. (2006). *Managing to nurse: Inside Canada's health care reform.* University of Toronto Press.

Reed, P. (1995). A treatise on nursing knowledge development for the 21st century: Beyond postmodernism. *Advances in Nursing Science, 17*(3), 70–84.

Risjord, M. (2010). *Nursing knowledge: Science, practice, and philosophy.* Wiley-Blackwell.

Rolfe, G. (2000). *Research, truth, and authority: Postmodern perspectives on nursing.* Macmillan Press.

Roy, C., Sr., & Jones, D. A. (Eds.). (2007). *Nursing knowledge development and clinical practice.* Springer Publishing Company.

Rudge, T. (2013). Desiring productivity: Nary a wasted moment, never a missed step! *Nursing Philosophy, 14*(3), 201–211.

Sandelowski, M. (1999). Troubling distinctions: A semiotics of the nursing/technology relationship. *Nursing Inquiry, 6*(3), 198–207.

Sandelowski, M. (2000a). *Devices and desires: Gender, technology, and American nursing.* University of North Carolina Press.

Sandelowski, M. (2000b). Paradigms and presuppositions: The difference between qualitative and quantitative research. *Scholarly Inquiry for Nursing Practice, 14*(2), 157–160.

Sandelowski, M. (2002). Visible humans, vanishing bodies, and virtual nursing: Complications of life, presence, place, and identity. *Advances in Nursing Science, 24*(3), 58–70.

Sokal affair. (2022, February 2). In *Wikipedia.* https://en.wikipedia.org/wiki/Sokal_affair

Soper, K. (1986). *Humanism and anti-humanism.* Hutchinson.

Thompson, J. L. (1998). Response to Drevdahl. *Scholarly Inquiry for Nursing Practice, 12*(4), 319–323.

Thompson, J. L. (2007). Poststructuralist feminist analysis in nursing. In Sr. C. Roy & D. A. Jones (Eds.), *Nursing knowledge development and clinical practice* (pp. 129–144). Springer Publishing Company.

Thompson, J. L., Allen, D. G., & Rodriguez-Fisher, L. (Eds.). (1992). *Critique, resistance, and action: Working papers in the politics of nursing.* NLN.

Tomey, A. M., & Alligood, M. R. (Eds.). (2006). *Nursing theorists and their work* (6th ed.). Mosby.

Traynor, M. (2006). Discourse analysis: Theoretical and historical overview and review of papers in the Journal of Advanced Nursing 1996–2004. *Journal of Advanced Nursing, 54*(1), 62–72.

Walter, S. (2011, October 11). The myth of American exceptionalism. *Foreign Policy.* https://foreignpolicy.com/2011/10/11/the-myth-of-american-exceptionalism/

Watson, J. (1995). Postmodernism and knowledge development in nursing. *Nursing Science Quarterly, 8*(2), 60–64.

Watson, J. (1999). *Postmodern nursing and beyond.* Churchill Livingstone.

Appendix

Table A1 American Postmodern, Post-structural, and Foucauldian Field: Articles by American Nurses (and Non-American Nurses in American ANS) Referring to Postmodernism, Post-structuralism, or Foucault from the Late 1980s to the End of 2010
  Abbreviations used:

ANS: *Advances in Nursing Science*
AJCC: *American Journal of Critical Care*
IMHN: *Issues in Mental Health Nursing*
JAN: *Journal of Advanced Nursing*
JNE: *Journal of Nursing Education*
NAQ: *Nursing Administration Quarterly*
NI: *Nursing Inquiry*
NP: *Nursing Philosophy*
NSQ: *Nursing Science Quarterly*
PHN: *Public Health Nursing*
RTNP: *Research and Theory for Nursing Practice*
SINP: *Scholarly Inquiry for Nursing Practice*

(A) Textbooks that anthologize a given paper
(S) Summary for selected articles, primarily those not mentioned in the chapters

All <u>non-American entities are underlined</u> (i.e. non-American journals and anthologies and articles in American journals authored by non-American nurses)

Year from the earliest	Author, title, journal Whether anthologized (A) and a brief summary (S) <u>Non-American authors and sources underlined</u>
1. 1989	Dzurec L. The necessity for and evolution of multiple paradigms for nursing research: A poststructuralist perspective. ANS A: Omery, Kasper, & Page (1995) *In search of nursing science.* (An original chapter) A: Polifroni & Welch (1999) *Perspectives on philosophy of science in nursing.*

(Continued)

(Continued)

Year from the earliest	Author, title, journal Whether anthologized (A) and a brief summary (S) <u>Non-American authors and sources underlined</u>
2. 1990	Dickson G. L. A feminist poststructuralist analysis of the knowledge of menopause. ANS A: Chinn (1994) *Developing nursing perspectives in women's health*. ANS Series.
3. 1992	Doering L. Power and knowledge in nursing: A feminist poststructuralist view. ANS
4. 1995	Watson J. Postmodernism and knowledge development in nursing. NSQ A: Chaska (2001) *The nursing profession: Tomorrow and beyond.* (An original chapter) A: Polifroni & Welch (1999) *Perspectives on philosophy of science in nursing.*
5. 1995	Henneman E. Nurse–physician collaboration: A poststructuralist view. <u>JAN</u> S: In this article by a nurse and doctoral student from University of California, Los Angeles, Henneman identifies her research interest in the phenomenon of nurse–physician collaboration and justifies her interest in this topic and in the "practical issues related to patient care" (p. 363), making the article a justificatory argument. Running through Henneman's argument is a thread about the American nursing theory movement engrossed in attempts to find the "unique nursing paradigm," which grants legitimacy to writings that oppose medicine and medical science (i.e., "the positivist model" maligned in nursing). Henneman implicitly raises a question: Where does (academic) nursing's position leave nurses on the hospital floor whose practice is inextricably defined by their relations with physicians and others? The author's epiphany is a call for pluralism—the coexistence of medical science and nursing science—that will open discussions of professional interdependence. She advocates "multiple paradigms" (p. 361), using Foucault as a rhetorical leverage to advocate multiple "ways of knowing" and methods of inquiry. Foucault helped to restore the "pluralism" inclusive of medicine and physicians as part of the health care team.
6. 1995	Reed P. A treatise on nursing knowledge development for the 21st century: Beyond postmodernism. ANS A: Polifroni & Welch (1999) *Perspectives on philosophy of science in nursing.* A: Reed & Shearer (2009) *Perspectives on nursing theory.*
7. 1996	Koerner J. G. Imagining the future for nursing administration and systems research. NAQ A: <u>Rolfe (2000) Research, truth, authority</u>. S: Koerner discusses postmodernism in terms of a "postmodern world-view" contrasted with a "modern world-view." The latter is represented by reductive, behaviourist sciences, whereas the former is described as a holistic science (including chaos theory, ecological Christianity, quantum physics). The simultaneity paradigm of nursing science (i.e., theories of Rogers, Newman, and Parse) is said to incorporate postmodern principles.
8. 1996	Powers P. Discourse analysis as a methodology for nursing inquiry. <u>NI</u>

Year from the earliest	Author, title, journal Whether anthologized (A) and a brief summary (S) <u>Non-American authors and sources underlined</u>
9. 1997	<u>Falk Rafael A. R.</u> Advocacy oral history: A research methodology for social activism in nursing. *ANS*
10. 1997	LeBlanc R. Definitions of oppression. <u>*NI*</u>
11. 1998	Drevdahl D. Diamond necklaces: Perspectives on power and the language of "community." *SINP*
12. 1998	<u>Glass N. & Davis K.</u> An emancipatory impulse: A feminist postmodern integrated turning point in nursing research. *ANS*
13. 1998	Johnson M. E. Being restrained: A study of power and powerlessness. *IMHN*
14. 1999	Drevdahl D. Meanings of community in a community health center. *PHN*
15. 1999	Bent K. Seeking the both/and of a nursing research proposal. *ANS*
16. 1999	Drevdahl D. Sailing beyond: Nursing theory and the person. *ANS*
17. 1999	Hall J. Marginalization revisited: Critical, postmodern, and liberation perspectives. *ANS*
18. 1999	Gadow S. Relational narrative: The postmodern turn in nursing ethics. *SINP* A: Kenney (2002) *Philosophical and theoretical perspectives for advanced nursing practice.* A: Cody (2006) *Philosophical and theoretical perspectives for advanced nursing practice.* A: Reed & Shearer (2009) *Perspectives on nursing theory.* S: A nurse with a background in German dialectic philosophy, Gadow describes nursing ethics as being inadequately conceived through two common approaches: (1) an account of "ethical immediacy" with "subjective certainty" guaranteed by the immersion into a supposedly organic tradition or community, and (2) an account of "ethical universalism" with "objective certainty" assured through the rational, detached appeal to principles and codes. In contrast, postmodern ethics embrace contingency, refuse certainties, and resist the drive for unity and foundations. Gadow cites Bauman on postmodern ethics; Foucault; and postmodern feminist writers Benhabib, Cixous, and Young.
19. 2000	Gadow S. Philosophy as falling: Aiming for grace. <u>*NP*</u>
20. 2000	David B. A. Nursing's gender politics: Reformulating the footnotes. *ANS*
21. 2001	Allen D. & Hardin P. Discourse analysis and the epidemiology of meaning. <u>*NP*</u>
22. 2001	Hardin P. Theory and language: Locating agency between free will and discursive marionettes. <u>*NI*</u>
23. 2001	Ironside P. Creating a research base for nursing education: An interpretive review of conventional, critical, feminist, postmodern, and phenomenologic pedagogies. *ANS*

(Continued)

(Continued)

Year from the earliest	*Author, title, journal* *Whether anthologized (A) and a brief summary (S)* <u>*Non-American authors and sources underlined*</u>
24. 2001	Phillips D. Methodology for social accountability: Multiple methods and feminist, poststructural, psychoanalytic discourse analysis. ANS
25. 2002	Arslanian-Engoren C. Feminist poststructuralism: A methodological paradigm for examining clinical decision-making. <u>JAN</u>
26. 2002	Watson J. & Smith M. Caring science and the science of unitary human beings: A trans-theoretical discourse for nursing knowledge development. <u>JAN</u>
27. 2002	Drevdahl D. Home and border: The contradictions of community. ANS
28. 2002	Thompson J. Which postmodernism? A critical response to Therapeutic touch and postmodernism in nursing. <u>NP</u>
29. 2002	Mitchell G. & Cody W. Ambiguous opportunity: Toiling for truth of nursing art and science. NSQ

Critical & postmodern perspectives. Chinn P. L., journal editor, *Advances in Nursing Science*, thematic journal issue (Includes articles 30–34 in the following list)

30. 2003	Hardin P. Social and cultural considerations in recovery from anorexia nervosa: A critical poststructuralist analysis. ANS
31. 2003	Phillips D. & Drevdahl D. "Race" and the difficulties of language. ANS
32. 2003	<u>Kushner K. & Morrow R.</u> Grounded theory, feminist theory, critical theory: Toward theoretical triangulation. ANS
33. 2003	Georges J. An emerging discourse: Toward epistemic diversity in nursing. ANS
34. 2003	Dzurec L. Poststructuralist musings on the mind/body question in health care. ANS
35. 2003	Hardin P. Shape-shifting discourses of anorexia nervosa: Reconstituting psychopathology. <u>NI</u>
36. 2003	Hardin P. Constructing experience in individual interviews, autobiographies and on-line accounts: A poststructuralist approach. <u>JAN</u>
37. 2003	Powers P. Empowerment as treatment and the role of health professionals. ANS
38. 2003	SmithBattle L. Displacing the "rule book" in caring for teen mothers. PHN
39. 2003	Cotton A. The discursive field of web-based health research: Implications for nursing research in cyberspace. ANS
40. 2003	Kendall J., Hatton D., Beckett A., & Leo M. Children's accounts of attention-deficit/hyperactivity disorder. ANS
41. 2004	Georges J. & McGuire S. Deconstructing clinical pathways: Mapping the landscape of health care. ANS
42. 2004	Reinhardt A. Discourse on the transformational leader metanarrative or finding the right person for the job. ANS
43. 2004	<u>Glass N. & Davis K.</u> Reconceptualizing vulnerability: Deconstruction and reconstruction as a postmodern feminist analytical research method. ANS

Year from the earliest	Author, title, journal Whether anthologized (A) and a brief summary (S) <u>Non-American authors and sources underlined</u>
44. 2004	Benner P. Seeing the person beyond the disease. AJCC
45. 2004	Soltis-Jarrett V. Interactionality: Willfully extending the boundaries of participatory research in psychiatric-mental health nursing. ANS
46. 2005	Allen D. & Cloyes K. The language of "experience" in nursing research. <u>NI</u>
47. 2005	Phillips D. Reproducing normative and marginalized masculinities: Adolescent male popularity and the outcast. <u>NI</u>
48. 2005	Georges J. Linking nursing theory and practice: A critical-feminist approach. ANS
49. 2005	Kramer M. Self-characterizations of adult female informal caregivers: Gender identity and the bearing of burden. <u>RTNP</u>
50. 2006	Allen D. Whiteness and difference in nursing. <u>NP</u>
51. 2006	<u>Ogle K. R. & Glass N.</u> Mobile subjectivities: Positioning the nonunitary self in critical feminist and postmodern research. ANS
52. 2006	Cloyes K. G. An ethic of analysis: An argument for critical analysis of research interviews as an ethical practice. ANS
53. 2006	Cloyes K. Prisoners signify: A political discourse analysis of mental illness in a prison control unit. <u>NI</u>
54. 2006	Tinley S. T. & Kinney A. Y. Three philosophical approaches to the study of spirituality. ANS
55. 2008	Campesino M. Beyond transculturalism: Critiques of cultural education in nursing. JNE
56. 2009	SmithBattle L. Pregnant with possibilities: Drawing on hermeneutic thought to reframe home-visiting programs for young mothers. <u>NI</u>
57. 2009	Lagerwey M. D. In their own words: Nurses' discourses of cleanliness from the Rehoboth Mission. <u>NI</u>
58. 2010	Kagan P., Smith M., Cowling W. I., & Chinn P. A nursing manifesto: An emancipatory call for knowledge development, conscience, and praxis. <u>NP</u>
59. 2010	Nosek M., Kennedy H., & Gudmundsdottir M. Silence, stigma, and shame: A postmodern analysis of distress during menopause. ANS
60. 2010	Kako P. M. & Dubrosky R. "You comfort yourself and believe in yourself": Exploring lived experiences of stigma in HIV-positive Kenyan women. *IMHN* S: The authors draw on Goffman's notion of stigma and Foucault's notion of heterotopia ("the societal process of stigmatization in creation of other spaces," those of deviance and of crisis, p. 151).
61. 2010	Kagan P. N. & Chinn P. L. We're all here for the good of the patient: A dialogue on power. NSQ
62. 2010	Polifroni E. C. Power, right, and truth: Foucault's triangle as a model for clinical power. NSQ

Table A2 American Postmodern, Post-structural, and Foucauldian Field (continued): References to Postmodernism, Post-structuralism, and Foucault in American Nursing Textbooks

Abbreviations used:

ANS: *Advances in Nursing Science*
JAN: *Journal of Advanced Nursing*
NI: *Nursing Inquiry*
NP: *Nursing Philosophy*
SINP: *Scholarly Inquiry for Nursing Practice*

Part One. Long-running editions of nursing theory textbooks (in alphabetical order based on the first author)

1.1
Chinn P. L. & Jacobs M. K. (1983) *Theory and nursing: A systematic approach.*
1987 – 2nd ed.
Chinn P. L. & Kramer M. K. (1991) *Theory and nursing: A systematic approach.* 3rd ed.
1995 – 4th ed.
1999 – *Theory & nursing: Integrated knowledge development.* 5th ed.
2004 – *Integrated knowledge development in nursing.* 6th ed.
2008 – *Integrated theory and knowledge development in nursing.* 7th ed.
2011 – 8th ed.
Beginning with early editions, this book is structured on Carper's (1978) patterns of knowing, modified and extended by Chinn. In Chinn and Kramer's (e.g. 1999) framework of "integrated knowledge development," the notion of *theory* (and an extensive elaboration of nature, structure, and validation strategies of theory, as well as the role of research and practice for theory generation and testing) is affiliated squarely with "empiric knowledge," that is, "the use of sensory experience for creation of mediated knowledge expressions" (p. 253). The other three "patterns of knowing" – ethical, personal, and aesthetic – much valued by the authors, are discussed in separate chapters but *not* in any way associated with *theory*. The Table of Contents clearly structures the domains of knowledge and rhetorically places the notion of theory exclusively within one of them. The significance for my argument of such classificatory practices lies in channelling the reader's vision and allowing some phenomena to be perceived in particular ways while others are obscured. (My own attempt to recast and reconfigure the body of Foucauldian nursing scholarship is no exception.) Chinn and Kramer's text, as do many other nursing theoretical sources, identifies some nurse scholars as theorists and others as ethicists. Most notably, American nurse scholars Joan Liaschenko (who studied morality of nursing practice) and Margarete Sandelowski (who wrote on the aesthetics of qualitative research), both favourably cited by Chinn and Kramer (1999, 2011), have been "locked" in the domains of "ethical knowledge" (as has been another American scholar, Sally Gadow, by other commentators) and of "aesthetics," respectively. Unwittingly, the framework of "integrated knowledge development" effectively decouples the highly theoretical scholarship of these three scholars from the realm of "theory" in the discourse of nursing knowledge. Non-American postmodern and post-structural nurse authors are similarly screened out by such a framework.

Starting with the sixth edition, Chinn and Kramer (2004) acknowledge, over two pages, "emerging trends of knowledge development" (p. 38) comprised of "interpretive and critical approaches" and "poststructuralist approaches." Varieties of critical theory are summarized thus: "Critical feminist theory centers on issues of gender discrimination. Critical social theory focuses on class issues as they perpetuate unfair educational, political, and other social practices. The 'critical' focus points to a need to undo and remake oppressive social structures" (p. 40). A paragraph on postmodernism indicates the term's lack of clarity and a postmodern de-centring of the scientific method with acceptance of various research methods. A one-page subsection on "poststruturalist approaches" cites Allen and Hardin (2001) in *NP*; Francis (2000) in *NI*; and Arslanian-Engoren (2002) in *JAN*. A paragraph on poststructuralism ends with the following synopsis: "Critical language and discourse analyses that uncover how language functions to perpetuate systems of oppressions and domination are important new dimensions to nursing knowledge" (p. 40).

The eighth edition (Chinn & Kramer, 2011) has two notable features:

1 A half-page section on "poststructuralist approaches" (p. 51) cites Cloyes (2006) in *ANS*; Thompson (2007) in Roy and Jones; Tinley and Kinney (2007) in *ANS*, in addition to those papers listed before. Post-structuralism is described as before. A new separate half-page section on "deconstruction and postmodernism" (p. 51) is added. Postmodernism is described as before. Deconstruction is said to involve analyses of texts (written, visual) to uncover assumptions, ideologies, and frames of reference and to show them as unwarranted bases for truths. The goal of deconstruction is to undermine unjust language and social practices (p. 51).

Of interest to me is that within this chapter's discussion of evidence-based practice (EBP), three other articles are cited (all by non-American nurses) that are informed by postmodernism/post-structuralism: Evans, Pereira and Parker (2009) in *NI* on the dominant role of medicine in directing nursing practice; Rolfe (2006) in *NI* on the clinical relevance of theory and research; and Holmes, Perron and O'Byrne (2006) on the critique of EBP. It appears as though Chinn and Kramer do not acknowledge these articles as *examples* of postmodern/post-structural nursing work (i.e., as applications of postmodern and post-structural ideas to analyse nursing issues).

2 A novel feature of this edition is a newly formulated pattern of knowing, "emancipatory, or the praxis of nursing," central to and interrelated with the other four. A separate chapter devoted to emancipatory knowing outlines its three facets: Habermas's three fundamental human interests (technical, practical, and emancipatory); Freire's liberation theory; and the poststructuralism of Foucault (p. 71). It is noteworthy that post-structuralism is said to be "anti-realist."

In this long-running textbook, postmodernism and post-structuralism are selectively "noticed" when they are useful to counter "oppression and domination," the title includes keywords (e.g. "Feminist poststructuralism: A methodological paradigm for examining clinical decision-making" by Arslanian-Engoren, 2002), and the authors are American nurses. Thus, the book adopts an "additive" approach to knowledge: The rest of the book's ideas are immune to postmodern and post-structural challenges.

1.2

Fawcett J. (2005) *Contemporary nursing knowledge: Analysis and evaluation of nursing models and theories*. 2nd ed.

No references to postmodernism, post-structuralism, or Foucault based on my review of the table of contents and detailed index.

(*Continued*)

(Continued)

1.3

Fitzpatrick J. J. & Whall A. L. (1983) *Conceptual models of nursing: Analysis and application.*
1989 – 2nd ed.
2004 – 4th ed.
2016 – *Conceptual models of nursing: Global perspectives.* 5th ed.
Second edition: No references to postmodernism or post-structuralism.
Fifth edition: In her chapter "Philosophy of Science Positions and Their Importance in Cross-National Nursing," Whall (2016) devotes one page to a discussion of postmodernism. The basis of her discussion is Reed's (1995) article, which positions postmodernism as a stage in the philosophy of science following positivism and leading to a more desirable worldview of neomodernism (pp. 13–14).

1.4

Johnson B. M. & Webber P. B. *An introduction to theory and reasoning in nursing.*
2005 – 2nd ed.
2010 – 3rd ed.
The third edition is described as "presenting a detailed discussion of the relationship between theory, research, and reasoning in nursing" (Novak, 2010, p. xi). Some chapter titles are "Language, Meaning, and Structure"; "Theory and Reasoning"; "Foundations of Nursing Theory"; "Introduction to Research"; "Theory and Practice"; "Multidisciplinary Theory."
Although the authors are critical towards selected ideas from the American nursing metatheoretical literature (e.g. the four metaparadigm concepts, Parse's exotic language, or the idea that nursing theory should be completely isolated from "support theories" drawn from other disciplines), their presentation of theory reflects the logical positivist philosophy of science, as described by Risjord (2010). The most illustrative case of positivist influences is the authors' view of theory as consisting of "building blocks," starting from "observation of phenomena," and progressing upward through "ideas," "concepts," and "propositions." If these initial formulations are supported through research, that is, verified empirically, they become "facts, principles, and laws" of "established theories" (p. 23). The authors approvingly cite a 1971 *Primer in Theory Construction* by Reynolds; they also turn to Hempel's 1965 book as an authority on the nature of scientific laws.
Quite literally, Foucauldian ideas are unintelligible when approached from the framework of this book. The authors cite Holmes and Gastaldo's (2002) "Nursing as means of governmentality." The context for the discussion is Johnson and Webber's advocacy for the idea of "nursing laws," and Orem's self-care theory is suggested as one such law (pp. 29–30). Holmes and Gastaldo's work is read as supporting the universality of Orem's ideas and "nursing's focus on helping people care for themselves" (p. 30). Johnson and Webber write, "In 2002, when discussing governmentality and nursing's role in public policy, Holmes and Gastaldo highlighted the role nursing played in bringing the importance of self-care and self-responsibility to the forefront of socially responsible policy" (p. 30). Holmes and Gastaldo's attempt to interrogate nursing's unacknowledged role as an agent of biopolitics is transformed into a self-congratulatory narrative of nursing influencing public policy and deployed to support the "law" of unique nursing science.

The "Introduction to Research" chapter by Clarke (2010, pp. 217–249) mentions postmodernism when presenting the relationship between "philosophies and methodologies": Modernism is said to correspond to quantitative ("logical positivism/empiricism") methodology; postmodernism to qualitative methodology; and neomodernism to "undiscovered methods" ("futuristic existentialism"). This two-page discussion draws heavily on "postmodern" nursing metatheory by Reed (2009 [*sic*] 1995) and Watson (1999), before embarking on a standard, social science introduction to types of research and research process. Intriguingly, Cheek's (2000) *Postmodern and Post-structural Approaches to Nursing Research* is cited in the section on neomodernism. Contrary to what might be expected, postmodernism neither informs the chapter on language and meaning nor appears in the chapter on multidisciplinary theory.

The book has an important goal – develop clinical reasoning in nurses – and several examples, cases, and exercises in the text are geared towards this goal. At a glance, the authors draw on some valuable resources on critical thinking, for example, the 1995 MIT book *Cognition on Cognition*. However, synthesizing these sources with American nursing (meta)theory that unwittingly propagates a logical positivist conception of theory, the book's attempt to present a contemporary understanding of the processes of thinking and reasoning is obscured.

1.5

Kenney J. W. (1996) *Philosophical and theoretical perspectives for advanced nursing practice.*
1999 – 2nd ed.
2002 – 3rd ed.
Cody W. K. (2006) *Philosophical and theoretical perspectives for advanced nursing practice.*
    4th ed.
The third and fourth editions include Gadow's (1999) "Relational narrative: The postmodern turn in nursing ethics" article in a book section devoted to "nursing's metaparadigm of nursing and health." (Refer to Table 1A for article summary.)

1.6

Kim H. S. & Kollak I. (Eds.) (1999). *Nursing theories: Conceptual and philosophical foundations.*
2006 – 2nd ed.
This edited collection consisting of 16 chapters is unusual in the American nursing theoretical scene. First, it is truly international: co-edited by an American nurse metatheoretician (Kim) and a German nurse academic (Kollak). Only four contributors are Americans, including Kim and Powers, while the other nine are from Norway, Germany, and Sweden. Second, it is *the only* American textbook on the topic of nursing theory bringing together interdisciplinary perspectives from the fields of philosophy including continental, sociology, psychology, and gender studies. Third, it is *the only* American nursing theory textbook presenting sociological and continental-philosophical critical analyses of key American nursing theory. Finally, postmodernism, post-structuralism, and/or Foucault's work are confidently cited in some chapters.

1.7

Marriner A. (1986) *Nursing theorists and their work.*
Marriner Tomey A. (1989) 2nd ed.
1994 – 3rd ed.
Tomey A. & Alligood M. R. (1998) 4th ed.
2002 – 5th ed.
2006 – 6th ed.
Alligood M. R. & Tomey A. (2010) 7th ed.

(Continued)

(Continued)

Up to and inclusive of the fourth edition: No reference to nursing theoretical work informed by postmodern or post-structural theory.

Fifth edition: One of the introductory chapters, titled "History and Philosophy of Science," under the subheading *Emergent Views of Science and Theory in the Late 20th Century*, briefly summarizes Foucault's *The Order of Things*; however, no connection is made between this summary and the content of the chapter as well as the subject of nursing theory.

Sixth edition: In addition to a reference to Foucault as in the previous edition, his work is named among several philosophical influences on a "philosophy of caring" articulated by a Norwegian nurse and philosopher Kari Martinsen (pp. 167, 174). The episteme (conditions of possibility for knowledge) and de-centring of the subject are Foucault's themes said to influence Martinsen's work.

1.8

Meleis A. I. (1985) *Theoretical nursing: Development and progress.*

1991 – 2nd ed.

1997 – 3rd ed.

2007 – 4th ed.

2012 – 5th ed.

In the third edition, Meleis (1997) discusses the emergence, in the latter half of the 1980s, of "alternative approaches to knowledge" such as critical theory and feminism as a milestone of theoretical nursing. Meleis emphasizes that "such frameworks . . . maintained the integrity of the basic ontological beliefs that have historically guided nursing practice, for example, holism, integrated responses, and relationship with environment" (p. 45). Another part of the book presents three "perspectives on knowing": empiricist, feminist, and critical theory. In contrast with Chinn's writings on feminism that expose male domination and advocate for women's bonding, Meleis's notion of feminism reflects attention to gender in the sense of promoting "gender-sensitive theories" and affirming gender equity (p. 154). Critical theory, exemplified by the philosophy of Habermas and work of David Allen in nursing, focuses on power and emancipation. Again, Meleis finds it important to remind nurses that "critical theory is not a substitute for nursing theory" (p. 157). Similarly, the second edition addresses feminism and critical theory in this way.

Meleis's books are impressive: 600–800-page narratives of "theoretical nursing." A curious feature of these books is the last part, "Our Historical Literature" (e.g. Meleis, 2007). Comprising about one-third of the book's volume, this part includes a meticulous annotated bibliography of metatheoretical nursing literature from 1960 to1984 and a bibliography (citations) of theory and metatheory (the latter seems to be updated for each edition). A comparison of bibliographic sources in the third (1997) and fifth (2012) editions yields an interesting perspective on what an influential American nurse theorist considers worth mentioning as examples of nursing theory.

The third edition is silent on postmodernism, post-structuralism, and Foucault, although the bibliography includes Reed's (1995) and Watson's (1995) papers on postmodernism.

Starting with the fourth edition in 2007, the terms *postmodernism, post-structuralism,* and *postcolonialism* find their place in the text. What in the previous edition was presented as the three perspectives on knowing (i.e., empiricist, feminist, and critical theory) is expanded here into "four views of knowing" (p. 489) or "views of science" (p. 492): the received view; perceived view; interpretive view (encompassing "feminist knowing" and "critical knowing"); and "postmodernism, poststructuralism, and postcolonialism views." The latter is discussed over one-and-a-half pages and summarized in two tables. Meleis (2007) is possibly the only American nurse theorist who uses Drevdahl's (1999) paper as an example of post-structural critique of the notion of holistic person. Moreover, several articles informed by postmodernism and post-structuralism from *JAN, NI, NP,* and *ANS* are listed in the bibliography under critical theory and feminist perspectives. Meleis is also correct about post-structural anti-essentialism and its interest in "historicizing" various phenomena. Refreshingly, Meleis cites a few contemporary social theory texts. However, Meleis appears to be alarmed about nurses' interest in these intellectual movements. Her concern relates to an observation she makes that postmodernism "deconstructs concepts," structures, and metanarratives, as well as it expresses scepticism towards a project of "structured theoretical formulations" (pp. 496–497, 504), which she says is counterproductive to the processes of nursing knowledge development.

The fifth edition (2012) is similar in its presentation of postmodernism/post-structuralism in the body of the text. What is new in this edition is that Meleis takes a firm position towards postmodernism: "It failed to have a practical relevance for health problems within the field of medical sociology [she cites one non-nursing source here]. Similar assumptions could be made about its utility for nursing science" (p. 149). This section on postmodernism/post-structuralism/postcolonialism ends with the following cautionary note: "It is often said that all the 'post' epistemologies are all for 'everything goes' (Chinn & Kramer, 2003), and they do not allow for constructing and developing theories. Critics should continue to inform and challenge epistemic diversity for knowledge development in nursing" (p. 150).

The bibliography includes a range of citations to American and non-American postmodern and post-structural journal papers.

1.9
Nicoll L. H. (1986) *Perspectives on nursing theory.*
1992 – 2nd ed.
1997 – 3rd ed.
Shearer N. B. C., Nicoll L. H. & Reed P. G. (2004) 4th ed.
Reed P. G. & Shearer N. B. C. (2009) 5th ed.
The third edition of this anthology includes a paper by Gortner (1993) "Nursing's Syntax Revisited." This article dubs Foucault "a philosopher of the month" alongside Kuhn, Laudan, Habermas, and Toulmin.
The fifth edition of this anthology is comprised of 72 articles. Of the following ten articles eight cite/mention Foucault and/or postmodernism:
American participants of the nursing (meta)theoretical debates
1 Gortner (1993) – as before
2 Reed (1995) A treatise on nursing knowledge development for the 21st century. *ANS*
3 Whall & Hicks (2002) The unrecognized paradigm shift in nursing. *Nursing Outlook* (The authors invite nurses to recognize the shift in the philosophy of science from "positivism," which the authors associate with the medical model, to "neomodernism," associated, according to authors, with the work of Laudan and Lakatos published in 1977.)

(Continued)

(Continued)

American nurse "philosophers"/"ethicists"

4 Liaschenko & Fisher (1999) Theorizing the knowledge that nurses use in the conduct of their work. *SINP* (The authors do not draw on postmodern or post-structural ideas, but this work exemplifies interesting theorizing in our discipline, which however does not fit into the canon of American nursing theory.)

5 Gadow (1999) Relational narrative: The postmodern turn in nursing ethics. *SINP*

Non-American nurse authors

6 Nelson & Gordon (2004) The rhetoric of rupture. *Nursing Outlook* (This article does not cite Foucault, but reminds the reader that nursing is a *practice* with a history – an observation that challenges contemporary nursing discourses of professionalism, which operate ideologically by discounting nursing's past. That is, only the discipline of nursing – "unique nursing science" – is presented in American nursing theoretical literature as having a history, whereas nursing *practice* is ignored.)

7 Purkis & Bjornsdottir (2006) Intelligent nursing. *NP* (The authors extend postmodern theorizing of nursing practice by an Australian nurse J. Parker. Works of other social theorists, Giddens and Latour, also inform this analysis.)

8 Holmes & Gastaldo (2002) Nursing as means of governmentality. *JAN* (This analysis is based on Foucault's notions of power and governmentality, claiming nursing is a constitutive element of governmentality. The authors distinguish between "more oppressive and more caring" forms of governmentality constituting nursing practice, which differs from applications of the notion of governmentality by other Foucauldian scholars in nursing who are less sanguine about a "caring" form of governmentality.)

9 Rolfe (2006) Judgments without rules: Towards a postmodern ironist concept of research validity. *NI* (The author cites an array of French post-structural philosophers, Rorty, and American gurus of qualitative research Denzin and Lincoln.)

10 Stevenson & Beech (2001) Paradigms lost, paradigms regained: Defending nursing against a single reading of postmodernism. *NP* (The authors' thesis, as well as the sources they cite, echo Rolfe's ideas expressed in his book on postmodern nursing research.)

These last five articles approach nursing issues through a lens of contemporary continental philosophy. However, when these approaches are not explicitly signalled by the editors, but rather are assimilated within the framework of American nursing metatheory, this framework over-determines the potential readings of these pieces. One striking example is Johnson and Webber's interpretation of Holmes and Gastaldo (refer to point 1.4 listed earlier).

1.10
Parker M. E. (1993) *Patterns of nursing theories in practice.*
Parker M. E. (2006) *Nursing theories and nursing practice.* 2nd ed.
Parker M. E. & Smith M. C. (2010) 3rd ed.
No references to postmodernism, post-structuralism, or Foucault based on my review of the table of contents and detailed index.

1.11
Smith M. J. & Liehr P. R. (Eds.) (2003) *Middle range theory for nursing.*
2014 – 3rd ed.
No references to postmodernism, post-structuralism, or Foucault based on my review of the table of contents and index.

1.12
Walker L. O. & Avant K. C. (1983) *Strategies for theory construction in nursing.*
1995 – 3rd ed.
2005 – 4th ed.
2011 – 5th ed.
As the previous editions, the fifth edition begins with an overview of theory and
theory development in nursing. Describing the "evolution of theory development,"
the authors sketch, over two pages, how views of science and theory "expanded" in
the American nursing discipline, from criticisms of logical positivism to addition of
qualitative methodologies. The authors observe that from the mid-1980s and through
the 1990s, philosophical perspectives of critical theory and feminism have been
introduced into debates on nursing science. Summarizing the main points from the
paper by J. Campbell and Bunting (1991) "Voices and Paradigms: Perspectives on
Critical and Feminist Theory in Nursing" published in ANS, Walker and Avant devote
a paragraph each for critical theory and feminism. Then, the following paragraph
addresses postmodernism as it has emerged in nursing literature: as a challenge to
modern science and as an approach requiring caution.
The fourth edition presents postmodernism in the same way.
Of interest is that the authors set up a learning activity called "The disparagement of
20th-century nurse theorists." They set the stage with a comment about a common
rejection of nursing theory by students and nurses. To make students think about such
"unfair practices" (my words), the authors advise students to read Nelson and Gordon
(2004; anthologized in Reed & Shearer, 2009; and discussed earlier in point 1.9) and
to reflect upon some questions. The questions guide students to consider whether
nurse educators, when teaching courses on nursing theory, perhaps treat some nursing
theory without respect and express ad hominem attack towards selected theorists, and
whether, in general, past contributions of nurse theorists are undervalued.
It is ironic that, although Nelson and Gordon's main point is indeed a critique of the
subjugation of nursing's history in attempts to position current nursing as a radical
departure from the past, this critique is only a thinly veiled undermining of the
American nursing theory movement – including the very narrative presented by
Walker and Avant. Nelson and Gordon (2004) write: "In nursing, the profession and
its elites have a well-articulated history, but nursing practice does not. If a commonly
accepted discourse is blind to the skill and competence of ordinary nurses of the past,
it risks denying the skill and competence of ordinary nurses in the present" (p. 76). It
is curious but also perhaps illustrative that the intellectual matrix of American nursing
science instantiated in Walker and Avant's writing about nursing knowledge precludes
their interpretation of Nelson and Gordon as a *critique* of American nursing theory.

Part Two. Other American nursing textbooks (in chronological order)

2.1

Thompson J. L., Allen D. G. & Rodriguez-Fisher L. (Eds.) (1992) *Critique, resistance, and action: Working papers in the politics of nursing.*

Includes 12 papers presented at the second conference on Critical and Feminist Perspectives in Nursing in 1991 in Ohio.

(a) Allen in "Feminism, Relativism, and the Philosophy of Science" cites feminist philosophers, Foucault, Giddens, Rorty and others to present models of inquiry practised in the humanities that can be useful for nurses. This chapter is included in Rafferty and Traynor's (2002) book (Refer to Table A3).

(b) Thompson in "Identity Politics, Essentialism, and Constructions of 'Home' in Nursing" draws on anti-essentialist feminist writings participating in politics of difference to challenge "essentializing approaches to nursing identity" (p. 30).

(c) Maeda Allman in "Race, Racism, and Health: Examining the 'Natural' Facts" cites Haraway and Foucault.

2.2

Chinn P. L. (1994) *Advances in Nursing Science series.* Aspen Publishers.
  • *Developing nursing perspectives in women's health.*
  • *Advances in methods of inquiry for nursing.*

A series of thematic anthologies of selected articles published in *ANS*. One exception is *Advances in Methods of Inquiry*, which includes manuscripts submitted to *ANS* and selected by a peer review but not published due to a large volume of submissions for that particular issue. From the four volumes in this series that I accessed, three articles cite Foucault and other post-structural theorists.

Developing nursing perspectives in women's health.

(a) Dickson (1990) Feminist poststructuralist analysis of the knowledge of menopause.

Drawing on several works of Foucault and interviews with a group of women, the author illustrates how dominant societal discourses, that is, a biomedical view of menopause, shape women's perceptions of their bodies. This research is an early example of Foucault-informed analysis of interview texts, which tries to discern operations of power/knowledge in discourse.

Advances in methods of inquiry for nursing.

(a) Purkis (1994) Representations of action: Reorienting field studies in nursing practice.

This article by a Canadian nurse scholar is a critique of nursing field studies or ethnographies.

(b) Cheek & Rudge (1994) Inquiry into nursing as textually mediated discourse.

These Australian authors introduce a novel method of discourse analysis: "Language as a meaning-constituting system that is both historically and socially situated" (p. 59).

2.3

Omery A., Kasper C. E. & Page G. G. (Eds.) (1995) *In search of nursing science.*

Includes two chapters by L. Dzurec introducing post-structuralism and Foucault's power/knowledge.

2.4

Benner P. (Ed.) (1994) *Interpretive phenomenology: Embodiment, caring, and ethics in health and illness.*

Patricia Benner, an influential American nurse theorist known for formalizing the five stages of development of a nurse's competence from novice to expert and for proposing a methodology of interpretive phenomenology based on Heidegger's ideas, occasionally cites Foucault's *The Birth of the Clinic* (e.g. in her chapter in this book). However, with M. Heidegger, A. MacIntyre, and C. Taylor being the central influences, her use of Foucault is peripheral. In addition to being episodic, Benner's references to Foucault ignore his key insight about the operation of power. This omission results in descriptions of nursing practice that are naive and "evangelistic" in their treatment of power (Purkis, 1994).

2.5

Polifroni E. C. & Welch M. (1999) *Perspectives on philosophy of science in nursing: An historical and contemporary anthology.*

As the title conveys, philosophy of science is the unifying theme of this collection. Topics in philosophy of science (e.g. truth, explanation, science, and gender) and continental philosophical movements (e.g. phenomenology, critical theory, feminism, and postmodernism) are illustrated by a selection of nursing work. Among the advantages of this collection is inclusion of excerpts from original works by philosophers of science and continental philosophers.

Together with *In Search of Nursing Science* (Omery et al., 1995), this collection is one of the earliest American nursing metatheory texts that present a separate section on postmodernism.

The final section of the book, "Postmodernism and Nursing Science," includes three articles by Watson (1995), Reed (1995), and Dzurec (1989).

What limits the ability, in American nursing literature, to appreciate the full scope of postmodern and post-structural criticisms in philosophy and other humanities, is the lasting and confining enmeshment of ("legitimate") nursing theoretical scholarship with the notion of "nursing science." From a variety of post-structural writings available in *ANS* (not to mention *NI* and *JAN*) in the late 1990s, Polifroni and Welch select only the three aforementioned articles for their anthology. Of interest, too, is that no original philosophical work by French philosophers is included in this section.

In a brief introduction to this section, the editors describe what they see as the main postmodern ideas: the endorsement of multiple "approaches to knowledge," the relationship between power and knowledge theorized by Foucault, and Rorty's claim that "the concern for truth within postmodernism is replaced with a concern for meaning and utility."

Reviewing this book, Hussey (2001), who has a background in analytic philosophy, comments that some contemporary and valuable ideas in philosophy of science presented in this anthology are thoroughly buried within outdated and inaccurate ones; thus, in the absence of guidance, the reader is unlikely to separate the wheat from the chaff. This observation, I suggest, applies equally to the section on postmodernism.

2.6

Powers P. (2001) *The methodology of discourse analysis.*

Penny Powers completed her doctoral work at the University of Washington (supervisor D. Allen). In Chapter 5, I discuss a small group of American scholars mentored by Allen and/or participating in the conferences on Critical and Feminist Perspectives in Nursing, whom I call "the enclave group." Powers and other "enclave" scholars are among a few American nurse authors embracing Foucault's notion of discourse and using discourse analysis in their research.

2.7

Rodgers B. L. (2005). *Developing nursing knowledge: Philosophical traditions and influences.*

The advantage of this textbook is its focus on the development of nursing knowledge not limited to the canon of American nursing theory but attentive to nursing work informed by postmodernism, post-structuralism, hermeneutics, and critical theory. A chapter on the "postmodern turn" surveys key notions commonly associated with postmodern and post-structural movements and refers to the work of Foucault, Lyotard, and Derrida. Usefully, this survey goes into greater depth than other monographs on "nursing knowledge" such as Chinn and Kramer or Meleis. But even in Rodgers, interpretations of postmodernism and post-structuralism are usually limited to those accepted in American nursing theory literature: an emphasis on the criticism of the metanarrative of medical science and on the celebration of methodological pluralism including human sciences (nursing as a human science) and qualitative research (pp. 139–142).

(*Continued*)

(Continued)

The major limitation in how postmodernism and post-structuralism are presented relates to the book's framework that does not embed these movements in the context of continental philosophy, but rather in the context of selected ideas from the philosophy of science blended with the American philosophy of nursing science. It is these disciplinary traditions rather than the disciplinary lenses from the humanities that shape Rodgers's presentation of postmodernism and post-structuralism for nurses.

2.8

Dunphy L. & Longo J. (2007) Reflections on postmodernism, critical social theory, and feminist approaches: The postmodern mind. In P. L. Munhall (Ed.) *Nursing research: A qualitative perspective.* 4th ed.

Longo J. & Dunphy L. M. (2012) Postmodern philosophy and qualitative research. In 5th ed.

In the fifth edition, "traditional positivistic science" is contrasted with "critical science" said to encompass postmodernism, critical theory, and feminist theory. A brief summary of critical theory and feminism and their applications in nursing mostly draws on examples from *Advances in Nursing Science*. Following Chinn and Kramer, the authors characterize critical science as concerned with social justice. Postmodern research is discussed with reference to the work of P. Lather, an American education scholar who advocates freedom from rigid rules in inquiry (p. 106).

This chapter appeared first in the fourth edition and has been minimally revised since.

2.9

Thompson J. (2007) Poststructuralist feminist analysis in nursing. In C. Roy & D. A. Jones (Eds.) *Nursing knowledge development and clinical practice.*

Janice Thompson, one of the American "enclave" scholars during the 1990s (refer to Chapter 5), was later a nursing professor in a Canadian university. Her chapter presents a well-informed summary of postmodern and post-structural feminist theory. These ideas are then used to critique biomedical ethics as well as Benner's phenomenological analyses of nursing practice.

Papers in this collection, mostly by noted American nurse theorists and metatheoreticians (e.g. Roy, Chinn, Rodgers, Newman, Kim), were presented at New England Nursing Knowledge conferences.

2.10

Dahnke M. D. & Dreher H. M. (2011) *Philosophy of science for nursing practice: Concepts and application.*

This textbook, designed primarily for students in the Doctor of Nursing Practice (DNP) programs in the United States, brings together the perspectives of an author with a background in philosophy of science (Dahnke) and a nurse educator (Dreher).

Dahnke and Dreher distinguish between the philosophy of science and the philosophy of social science (postmodernism and Foucault are mentioned in both contexts) thus implying that "postmodernism" produced various influences and lends itself to various readings and various kinds of scholarly applications. Dahnke and Dreher's exposition is informed by philosophical sources rather than American nursing science writings. A persistent issue with the latter relates to a less-informed and often reified perception of science, philosophy, and interdisciplinary social theory in American nursing metatheory. Dahnke and Dreher, by the virtue of their education outside of the realm of American nursing theory (one in philosophy, the other in the *nursing practice* streams of American nursing education), avoid the pitfalls of purely nursing American textbooks that enthusiastically but mostly uncritically intermingle philosophy of science with "philosophy of nursing science and nursing theory" (see, e.g. Polifroni & Welch, 1999; Rodgers, 2005).

References to Foucault in Dahnke and Dreher include mentioning a sympathetic reading of Foucault's work by Ian Hacking, a contemporary philosopher of science, who suggests that what is socially constructed *exists* (contrary to accusations that Foucault denies reality).

This is one of few American nursing textbooks (alongside Kim and Kollak, the American "enclave" scholarship, and non-American Foucault-informed pieces in Shearer and Reed) that presents a good quality albeit brief summary of key postmodern and Foucault's notions such as metanarrative, knowledge/power, the panopticon, and antihumanism (p. 262). Regrettably, the authors focus on exposition of these ideas without any attempt to study their application in nursing in and outside of the United States.

Dahnke and Dreher, while presenting the philosophy of science in a well-informed manner, do not try to evaluate the philosophy of *nursing science* (i.e., nursing theory and metatheory). In contrast, a critical analysis of American nursing metatheory against a background of debates in philosophy of science is brilliantly done by Risjord (2010).

Table A3 Selected Non-American Foucauldian Field: Textbooks and Book Chapters by Non-American Authors (Nurses and Social Scientists Writing in Nursing) Citing Foucault from the Late 1980s to the End of 2015
Abbreviations used:

JAN: *Journal of Advanced Nursing*
NI: *Nursing Inquiry*
NP: *Nursing Philosophy*

Note: In contrast to the *American* postmodern, post-structural, and Foucauldian field up to approximately 2010 (including articles and books using these terms) captured in Tables A1 and A2, it would be nearly impossible to capture its *non-American* counterpart. The non-American postmodern, post-structural and Foucauldian field is vast: I estimate more than 700 articles published up to 2011, mostly in *NI*, *NP*, and *JAN*. This table captures only *books citing Foucault*. It includes neither occasional books exclusively using the terms *postmodernism* or *post-structuralism* nor *articles* citing any of these terms. Throughout the chapters, however, I cite diverse non-American postmodern, post-structural, and Foucauldian sources and focus on selected early examples.

This table also includes milestones in nursing continental-philosophical scholarship such as conferences and the formation of scholarly groups (not numbered in the table). The table lists only Anglophone sources and excludes nursing Foucauldian scholarship emerging from Brazil and Spain (see Gastaldo & Holmes, 1999, for references to some of these sources). Prolific authors like D. Holmes, Purkis, Rolfe, and Rudge have produced numerous chapters dispersed throughout literature beyond my present review. However, their central ideas are equally developed in those books and articles that *did* inform my analysis.

Date from the earliest	Author, title, summary
1.1988	Dingwall R., Rafferty A. M., & Webster C. *An introduction to the social history of nursing.* These British authors write the social history of general and psychiatric nursing, midwifery, and health-visiting in the United Kingdom from the 19th century to the late 20th century. To provide a broader context of societal trends, in a few passages the authors draw on selected ideas from Foucault such as disciplinary society and the rise of the clinic and psychiatry.

Date from the earliest	Author, title, summary

1988

In 1988, the Institute for Philosophical Nursing Research (IPNR; later Unit, uPNR) was established in the Faculty of Nursing, University of Alberta, under the leadership of Drs. June Kikuchi and Helen Simmons. From 1989, the Institute held biennial conferences in Banff, Alberta, Canada. The first IPNR conferences were invitational. Papers presented at the first three conferences, in 1989, 1991, and 1993, were published in three edited collections (Kikuchi & Simmons, 1992, 1994; Kikuchi, Simmons, & Romyn, 1996). At that time, conference attendees included mostly American nurse theorists and metatheoreticians. Although occasional references to postmodern and post-structural writers can be found in these collections, these are an exception. The Institute's early direction was significantly shaped by a conception of philosophy as metaphysics – a non-empirical search for the nature of nursing phenomena – and by the Institute's focus on American nursing (meta)theory rather than on continental philosophy and interdisciplinary social theory.

It is difficult to ascertain when and how Foucault "entered" the halls of the uPNR, but the three conferences I attended starting in 2010, have prominently featured postmodern and post-structural nursing theorizing.

2.1991 Lawler J. *Behind the screens: Nursing, somology, and the problem of the body.* A dissertation-based monograph by an Australian nurse and a sociologist. Theorizing findings of an ethnographic study, the author draws extensively on several of Foucault's books as well as other social theory.

3.1991 Gray G. & Pratt R. (Eds.) *Towards a discipline of nursing.* This Australian textbook consisting of 22 chapters is an introduction to the nursing profession for students in academic nursing programs. This first edition is written during the wave of reforms in nursing education in Australia that resulted in the transition of pre-licensure education of nurses from hospital schools of nursing into university departments. A remarkable feature of this book is contributors' references to continental philosophical literature (e.g. Habermas) as well as their familiarity with and variegated reception of American nursing theory from acceptance to questioning and rejection. Postmodernism, post-structuralism, and/or Foucault are referred to in seven chapters.

4.1992 Street A. F. *Inside nursing: A critical ethnography of clinical nursing practice.* A dissertation-based monograph by an Australian educator engaged in the higher education of nurses. This research was supervised and guided by American critical pedagogy scholars P. McLaren and H. Giroux. Of interest is the author's extensive reliance on Habermas's theory with its emancipatory focus, attenuated by Foucault's scepticism about a possibility of knowledge free of power. Street acknowledges the tension but admits that the emancipatory goal is hard to abandon. On pp. 99–113, Street exposes tensions between Habermas's and Foucault's thinking generally ignored in the American nursing literature, which unproblematically mixes and matches both authors as instances of a "critical theory paradigm."

1994

Nursing Inquiry journal launched, under the U.K. publisher and an Australian editor, Judy Parker. Sioban Nelson succeeded Parker in 1996.

(Continued)

(Continued)

Date from the earliest	Author, title, summary
5.1995	Porter S. *Nursing's relationship with medicine: A critical realist ethnography.* A dissertation-based monograph by a nurse sociologist from Ireland. Porter develops a Marxist analysis of the nursing profession with a focus on the economic basis and class structure of capitalism. Foucault's conception of power, cited only once, is depicted as inferior to that offered by the late Frankfurt school.
6.1995	Street A. F. *Nursing replay: Researching nursing culture together.* As in her 1992 book, the author draws on a range of Foucault's ideas related to the disciplinary society and the power/knowledge nexus.
1996	The first annual international nursing philosophy conference convened at Swansea University by U.K. scholar Steven Edwards.
7.1997	Lawler J. (Ed.) *The body in nursing.* A collection of ten essays by Australian nurses mostly associated, as faculty or doctoral students, with the University of Sydney or La Trobe University. Foucault is cited by seven contributors, including Judith Parker, Trudy Rudge, Pamela van der Riet, and Lawler herself. Foucault-informed articles by these authors appeared in nursing journals throughout the 1990s. Parker's chapter, a brief exposition of a theory of postmodernity and its implications for nursing, is reprinted in *A body of work* (Parker, 2004; see in the following). Lawler draws on Foucault's power/knowledge and "games of truth." In a Foucauldian sense, "truth" is "a function of the rules and principles of its production and inseparable from the discourses employed to communicate it" (Lawler, 1997, in Rafferty & Traynor, 2002, p. 169). Lawler exposes the limitations of scientific biomedical and economic "truths" for "knowing the body and embodiment," which she argues is the central concern for nursing practice. (Lawler's chapter is reprinted in *Exemplary research for nursing and midwifery* by Rafferty & Traynor, 2002, see in the following).
8.1997	Thorne S. & Hayes V. (Eds.) *Nursing praxis: Knowledge and action.* This collection, edited by Canadian nurses, includes three chapters of uneven quality drawing on Foucault: (1) American D. M. Trainor presents a confusing vision of "Enlightenment in nursing"; (2) American S. Miller presents a good overview of Foucault's key concepts and postmodern feminisms; and (3) Canadians J. McCormick and J. Roussy discuss what they call "a feminist poststructuralist orientation to nursing praxis."
9.1998	Edwards S. (Ed.) *Philosophical issues in nursing.* In a ten-chapter book, Foucault and other continental authors are cited in two chapters. American nurse Liaschenko uses the notion of clinical gaze when she describes the rise of modern scientific medicine. Australian nurse researcher Dawson advances a strong continentally informed critique of the notion of the self as an autonomous, rational, coherent, and agential consciousness, a view pervasive in ego-psychology and nursing, particularly in psychiatric nursing literature.

Date from the earliest	Author, title, summary
10.1998	Porter S. *Social theory and nursing practice.* A survey of sociological theory and its applications in nursing literature including • the three classics, E. Durkheim, K. Marx, and M. Weber; • symbolic interactionism, phenomenology, and ethnomethodology – perspectives focusing on individual action and the sociality of actions; • German critical theory and structuralism; • perspectives that bring together individual action and structure – Giddens's structuration theory and critical realism; • feminism; and • postmodernism. The last chapter, "Postmodernism and Foucault," depicts postmodernism as taking apart modernity's belief in rationality and progress. Porter explains Foucault's concepts of knowledge and discourse and illustrates them with an example of Cheek and Rudge's (1994) analysis of patient hospital records. Further, the concept of power is explained with references to panoptic surveillance, the clinical gaze, and pastoral power. This well-informed summary is accessibly written. Porter acknowledges his own allegiance to Habermas and a lukewarm perception of Foucault. In particular, Porter is critical of what he describes as Foucault's relativism (i.e., impossibility of a claim that one description of reality is better) and the latter's treatment of "reality as simply the creation of discourse" (p. 212). (Although such perceptions of Foucault are common, other commentators would disagree with Porter's assessment.)
11.1999	Clinton M. & Nelson S. (Eds.) *Advanced practice in mental health nursing.* Foucault is cited in two chapters: (a) Clinton and Nelson, both from Australia, argue that the historically contingent "understandings of *recovery* [from mental illness] delimit the therapeutic encounter and frame mental health nursing practice" (p. 260). If the prevalent images of mental health nursing posit the centrality of "humanistic and ontological concern for the patient" as in H. Peplau's vision (p. 273) or of patient empowerment (p. 274), in Clinton and Nelson's account, mental health nursing emerges as a "multiple . . . social form" (p. 260). Humanistic professional images of mental health nursing are shown to be not natural and universal but embedded in *societal* discursive framings of recovery. (b) Mason and Mercer, nurse academics from the University of Liverpool, describe the emergence of forensic psychiatric nursing.
12.1999	Robinson J., Avis M., Latimer J., & Traynor M. *Interdisciplinary perspectives on health policy and practice: Competing interests or complementary interpretations?*

(Continued)

(Continued)

Date from the earliest	Author, title, summary

The four British nurses (named before) have contributed two chapters each in addition to a co-authored introduction. Several chapters are of interest: (a) Avis, writing from a position of analytic philosophy and philosophy of science, refers to Foucault in the context of discussing epistemology as a branch of philosophy that addresses the nature of knowledge and of truth. Avis favours postmodern challenges to the foundationalism in science and to the primacy of the scientific method, especially Rorty's critiques of foundationalism. However, Avis rejects Lyotard's views on science as "epistemological relativism" (pp. 10–15; 89–92). (b) Traynor cites Foucault's *Discipline and Punish* in two chapters, "a literary approach to managerial discourse" (p. 119) and an examination of "morality and self-sacrifice in nursing talk" (p. 141). The latter chapter also provides background to the author's methodology – a post-structural approach to texts and discourse analysis. (c) Latimer, in her respective chapters, finds useful *The Birth of the Clinic* and the notion of governmentality.

13. 1999   Traynor M. *Managerialism and nursing: Beyond oppression and profession.*
A dissertation-based manuscript by a British nurse. The author has a background in English literature and employs literary theory and post-structural theorizing of language to analyse discourses of managerialism and professionalization shaping nursing practice.

14. 2000   Cheek J. *Postmodern and poststructural approaches to nursing research.*
A volume by an Australian sociologist whose articles, based on post-structural writers, frequently appeared in nursing journals during the 1990s. The book consists of chapters devoted to "postmodern thought" and the work of Foucault; "poststructural thought" and two "corresponding" approaches – discourse analysis and "deconstruction"; and "how to" illustrations (a research proposal and data tables) from a study conducted by the author on the media construction of toxic shock syndrome.

Cheek's overview of postmodernism and post-structuralism presents a particular "translation" of the theory, one that packages postmodern and post-structural ideas into an explicit qualitative research approach. She correctly identifies the difficulty of classifying Foucault's work, yet presents it as a postmodern theory. In turn, post-structuralism (exemplified by the writings of Derrida) is firmly tied to the notion of *text* in the following way: "The concept of text . . . is central to poststructural analysis and the concept of health care as textually mediated – that is, health care as shaped by and as shaping texts representing aspects of health care practices" (Cheek, 2000, p. 39). Arguably, rendering the notion of text in this specific way unwittingly moves "the text" and "practice" further apart rather than showing the benefits of conceiving of nursing practice itself as text (e.g. in a way that Judith Butler theorized gender as text in terms of gender's constitutive citationality). Shaping post-structural theory into an explicit "qualitative approach" aligns with a direction taken in some American social sciences in the early 1990s and led by Norman Denzin and his colleagues in their highly influential but problematic work on "qualitative paradigms."

Date from the earliest	Author, title, summary
15.2000	Latimer J. *The conduct of care: Understanding nursing practice.*

15.2000   Latimer J. *The conduct of care: Understanding nursing practice.*
A dissertation-based monograph by a British nurse with an English literature undergraduate education, later trained as a social scientist. The author describes her work as ethnography of the bedside based on H. Garfinkel's ethnomethodology with elements of discourse analysis and conversation analysis. As one of her analytical lines, Latimer argues that nurses develop "a particular form of nurse-patient relationship. . . . The patient has become the object of a nursing gaze, so the nurse conducts the [hospital] admission as if she is looking according to a grid of perceptions and then noting according to a code. But this conduct relays that neither the nurse nor the patient is a source of signification or legitimation; indeed, authority lies far from the bedside. This means that, in complete contrast to calls from theories of nursing [e.g. Benner], neither nurses nor patients author patients' needs" (p. 91). Foucault's notions of the clinical gaze and discourse underpin aspects of Latimer's analysis.

16.2000   Nelson S. *A genealogy of care of the sick.*
A dissertation-based monograph by an Australian nurse and a historian. Drawing on Mauss's notion of habitus and Foucault's *ethic of the self*, Nelson advances a powerful critique of holism in nursing as a valorized model of nurses' ethical comportment.

17.2000   Rolfe G. *Research, truth and authority: Postmodern perspectives on nursing.*
Gary Rolfe, a British nurse scholar and mental health/psychiatric nurse, first identifies his strong belief in the value of higher education for nurses. He invites nurses to read widely, especially in the humanities and summarizes "postmodern concepts of truth, science and research" (p. xiv) derived from Lyotard, Derrida, and Rorty to challenge what he calls modernist empirical research. Rolfe has selected five articles from nursing literature to illustrate "postmodern perspectives on nursing."
Rolfe draws on several Foucauldian ideas: the power/knowledge nexus; a discussion of the episteme of resemblance that characterized the Renaissance conception of truth (the unity between words and things), the episteme of representation in the Classical Age, and the episteme of self-reference characteristic of the modern age (a total break between words and things); and the regimes of truth.
Rolfe's discussion tends to present a simplistic image of modernist science and empirical research. Thus, on one side Rolfe places modernism, the Enlightenment project, positivism, traditional research approaches in sociology and psychology, technical rationality, and scientific method, all of which, according to the author, are based on a conception of a "single absolute truth." On the other side he places postmodern research with "a multitude of 'truths'" and "as many constructions of the truth as there are people in the world to construct it" (p. 3). He tackles the thorny issue of relativism often associated with postmodern views, advancing the possibility of a moral and epistemological stance that does not rely on the assumption of a "single truth" yet does not fall into a relativistic "abyss."

(Continued)

(Continued)

Date from the earliest	Author, title, summary
	A limitation of Rolfe's reading of postmodernism is encapsulated in the title of his chapter: "Postmodernism: The Challenge to Empirical Research." Rolfe's narrow understanding of "empirical research," equated with (post)positivist science and instrumental rationality, risks misrepresenting both empirical science and postmodern theory. His misrepresentation of science and the scientific method have garnered warranted corrections from, for example, Cave (1998) and Paley (2005), and his understanding of postmodernism screens out a possibility of empirical research, for instance, fieldwork or case studies, informed, methodologically and analytically, by postmodern thought. Rolfe's contribution to postmodern nursing scholarship lies in his ability to convey the *pleasure of text* (à la Barthes and Derrida) and in his persistence to demonstrate a relevance of the French literary theory for nursing.
2000	Seven attendees of the interdisciplinary conference on the topic of governmentality held in Finland organized into a group, *In Sickness & In Health* (aka *The Helsinki 7*). Sioban Nelson, associated with *Nursing Inquiry*, was one of the ISIH founding members, alongside British Anthony Pryce; Canadians Denise Gastaldo, Dave Holmes, and Mary Ellen Purkis; as well as Niels Buus from Denmark, and Kristin Bjornsdottir from Iceland. Subsequently, *Nursing Inquiry* published the conference papers presented by these nurses. The group later expanded. It organizes conferences where Foucault's ideas are still visible.
2000	*Nursing Philosophy* journal launched by a British publisher under the editorship of S. Edwards (the United Kingdom) and J. Liaschenko (the United States).
18.2002	Rafferty A. M. & Traynor M. (Eds.) *Exemplary research for nursing and midwifery.* A selection of 19 previously published research studies conducted by British, American, and Australian scholars (mostly nurses) from 1960 to 2000 and organized by the editors into three sections: "Research classics," "Conceptualising practice," and "Clinical effectiveness." The middle section, "Conceptualising practice," includes a number of papers relevant to my analysis. 1 A chapter by Lawler (1997) was addressed earlier. 2 Although T. Rudge, another nurse researcher engaged in ethnographic fieldwork, does not cite Foucault in this particular paper, she reads British and American anthropological methodological sources of the 1980s and 1990s that assimilated insights of postmodernism and post-structuralism. One of the central troubles with traditional empiricist ethnography is its "purported transparency and congruence with reality and experience," an assumption masking the role of language and writing in "invent[ing] culture" (Rudge, 1996, p. 157, in Rafferty & Traynor, 2002). In contrast, approaching ethnographic records as *text* reveals their perspectival and partial nature; these records are constructed narratives imbued with the (incoherent) subjectivities of the ethnographer.

Date from the earliest	*Author, title, summary*

3 An introduction by David Allen, an American nurse and women's studies scholar, to a book he co-edited (1992; Table A2 listed before). Allen's paper can be characterized as discursive – a term sometimes used in nursing literature to differentiate intellectual work not based on empirical findings, yet avoiding the label "philosophical" – in other words, a type of textual analysis common in the humanities. Allen considers the implications of recent philosophical ideas – communicative rationality articulated by Habermas, feminist philosophy of science, and Giddens's articulation of unintended consequences and unacknowledged conditions of human actions – for conceptualizations of research in the discipline of nursing.

An interesting feature of this book is its structure that helps to avoid two intractable issues. One issue is an American separation of the domain of theory (defined either as "nursing theory" or "borrowed theory") from the domain of research (unless research is firmly grounded in a clearly specified nursing theory). Rafferty and Traynor's perspective does not stem from such an understanding of nursing knowledge and thus avoids the theory/research binary (even if, undoubtedly, some studies foreground social theory while others foreground experimental method, these differences do not amount to the theory/research dualism).

The other issue, typical of nursing research textbooks (in particular, American and Canadian texts, with which I am most familiar), is a quantitative/qualitative division deepened by a further delineation of "research paradigms" in the context of the qualitative movement powerfully shaped by N. Denzin, Y. Lincoln, and E. Guba's writings (e.g. Denzin & Lincoln, 1994). Acknowledging the good intent and heuristic value of such classifications, leading nurse methodologists (e.g. Sandelowski) more recently have surfaced serious limitations accompanying the mainstream uptake of these classificatory schemas.

My exposure to vast nursing research literature leads me to similar conclusions: The limitations of accepted classifications pertain to the enduring tendency to formalize and then police "the research approaches" like "grounded theory" or "phenomenology" (mostly by extricating these "methodologies" from the ongoing practices of the social researchers). A twin tendency is to transform "paradigms" into incommensurable worldviews often used to attack the straw figures of "positivism" or "postmodernism," depending on the researchers' particular leanings.

(Continued)

(Continued)

Date from the earliest	Author, title, summary
19.2003	Latimer J. (Ed.) *Advanced qualitative research for nursing.*

This collection includes 12 chapters by researchers (mostly nurses) whose approaches to the study of nursing exhibit several important commonalities. First, all contributors skilfully draw on theory from different disciplines: anthropology, literary studies, history, sociology, and psychoanalysis. Second, the role of theory in research discussed by the contributors is such that it avoids a method/theory split. It is only possible for the researchers to reflect on their respective methodological decisions, analytical procedures, and outcomes in light of theoretical ideas guiding their interpretive efforts. That is, theory is not *applied* to a pre-established "qualitative" research methodology like "ethnography," "grounded theory," or "phenomenology." Rather approaches to research are designed along the lines of the disciplinary traditions (e.g. sociology, anthropology), taking into account contemporary theoretical debates in those disciplines. Next, all authors invite caution towards research accounts that naively or romantically privilege the constituting role of the human subject (patient, nurse, researcher) while ignoring the material, discursive, social, and historical constitution of human subjectivity. Consequently, nursing practice (and research practice) is approached as an inherently social process relying on relations among humans, material objects, and discursive formations. To take one example, Purkis posits "the radical separation between what nurses take to be their work and the actual work they are accomplishing" (p. 35). The relationship between a nurse and a patient then appears not as a self-evident fact but as "an active and knowledgeable social accomplishment" (p. 35).

Foucault is cited in six chapters: May problematizes evaluation research (ER) by showing how the use of qualitative ER can mask the power relations and surveillance in practices of evaluation. Savage and Latimer both cite *The Birth of the Clinic.* Traynor discusses an approach to discourse analysis informed by post-structural theory, which challenges the conception of language as a window onto either subjects' motivations or a reality free of ideology. Rather, Traynor views discourses "as enacting a desire for coherence, identity and solidarity partly through a connection to different historical projects . . . identification that can help to make the position and arguments of different groups more powerful" (p. 151). Rudge reflects on her discursive ethnographic study of nursing practice on a burn unit. She explores how "the various technologies intersect and interact to produce the wound care procedure as a spatio-temporal event" (p. 177) – the event where "nurses and patients are subjected to the powerful influences of scientific and relational discourses" and where they participate "in an ordering of knowledge(s) about wounds" (p. 178). Nelson criticizes conventional nursing historiographies based on a progressivist vision of history as the heroic achievements of enlightened individuals. To this, she contrasts other understandings of history attentive to "small" mundane activities and material implements used by nurses that reveal much about a largely unspoken world of nursing practice. Nelson also gives an example of Foucauldian genealogies, or histories of the present, that demonstrate socio-political contingencies of the "nursing breakthroughs."

Date from the earliest	Author, title, summary

2003

The International Philosophy of Nursing Society (IPONS) founded at the seventh nursing philosophy conference under the leadership of John Drummond and S. Edwards (the United Kingdom). The *Nursing Philosophy* journal becomes the official publication of the IPONS.

While Edwards is a philosopher educated in the analytic tradition, Drummond was a mental health nurse and a continentally orientated nurse philosopher whose highly respected work finds inspiration in Nietzsche, Deleuze, Lyotard, and the avant-garde movement.

Successful efforts to spearhead the domain of nursing philosophy in Canada (Kikuchi & Simmons, 1992, 1993) and in Britain (Edwards, 1998; Drummond & Standish, 2007) have relied on presenting philosophy as able to answer "questions that science cannot answer" (Kikuchi, 1992), that is, as a non-empirical endeavour concerned with metaphysics (Kikuchi, 2013) and ethics (Edwards, 1998), among philosophy's other concerns. Of course, actual scholarly practices of members of nursing philosophy groups span a wide range of approaches, including empirical studies. From its early days, the IPONS has encouraged philosophical work within both analytic and continental traditions, including critiques of Western metaphysics and ethics. Thus, in the discipline of nursing, postmodern and post-structural theory found its home in the nursing philosophy circles. However, the IPONS group has been diverse, with some members on occasion expressing a condescending attitude towards "postmodernism" (Hussey, 2004). In contrast, the *ISIH* group was formed on the basis of an explicit interest in Foucault's work without any overt connection to the field of philosophy.

20.2004	Freshwater D. & Rolfe G. *Deconstructing evidence based practice.* An experiment à la Derrida: a book with a (mis)placed beginning and end, intentionally without an index but with pages split into columns of (un)related texts and printed in mixed fonts. To dismantle EBP, the authors draw on the literary theory of Barthes, the philosophy of Derrida, a critique of the metanarrative of science by Lyotard, and selected ideas of Foucault. The publication of this book generated a reaction from its critics (e.g. Paley, 2005) and Rolfe's rejoinders (2005).
21.2004	Parker J. M. *A body of work: Collected writings on nursing.* This is a collection of selected conference papers and journal articles by an Australian nurse scholar. Parker (1997) theorized the body in nursing in light of postmodern criticisms of progressive history (futuristic temporality) and coherent subjectivity. Another theoretical influence on Parker's (Wiltshire & Parker, 1996) empirical studies of nursing practice is psychoanalytic theory, namely, Kristeva's concept of *abjection* and Bion's concept of *containing*. Parker (1980) reveals her sociological perspective that she explains as an attention to three dimensions of nursing – "the personal, the situational and the structural" (p. 260). I find striking Parker's (1986, 1989, 2000) ability to operate with the terminology of American nursing metatheory (e.g. unique nursing knowledge, basic nursing research, metaparadigm concepts, caring) but to skilfully re-populate these terms with drastically different meanings (e.g. the focus on the body, the non-romantic understanding of nurse–patient relationships, the role of technology, and a critical appraisal of American nursing models) thus undermining the familiar conceptions.

(*Continued*)

(Continued)

Date from the earliest	Author, title, summary

22.2006 Nelson S. & Gordon S. *The complexities of care: Nursing reconsidered.* Ten essays by authors from Australia, Canada, the United Kingdom, and the United States (mostly nurses but also a journalist, a sociologist, and a philosopher) all converge on a common goal – to challenge the "caring discourse" in nursing that romanticizes and oversimplifies knowledge and skills required by nurses in the complex realities of today's health care, including those instances of "emotional and relational care" valorized by the specifically constructed caring rhetoric in nursing. One of the issues with the caring discourse relates to its focus on nursing as an individualized art – a widespread view that disregards organizational and social factors shaping "care." Other concerns that the editors raise in the book are reflected in the emotionally laden and rhetorical questions: "So if RNs are supposed to be caring but have no time to care – to do emotional work – does that mean that they are not really authentic nurses? And if the nurses don't have time to do emotional work – and the rest of their work is invisible – have they failed? Are they no longer real nurses?" (Nelson & Gordon, 2006, p. 6). Foucault is alluded to in a chapter by Gordon, a journalist. Heartfield, an Australian nurse, turns to Foucault's notion of governmentality to analyse "the disappearance of patient recovery time" (p. 143) in surgical nursing.

23.2007 Drummond J. S. & Standish P. (Eds.) *The philosophy of nurse education.* The book consists of 12 chapters and a substantive introduction. References to Foucault appear in the text three times: (a) The introduction by a nurse philosopher from Scotland (Drummond) and a philosopher of education from Britain (Standish) provides a useful background to the (marginalized) place of philosophical inquiry in practice disciplines such as education and nursing. The main differences between the analytic and continental philosophical traditions are presented. (b) A chapter by an American educational psychologist Tina Besley, boldly titled "Foucault, Nurse Counselling and Narrative Therapy," presents the narrative approach to counselling (which, the author suggests, can be offered by nurses during their routine interactions with patients) as an alternative to the humanistic psychology of Carl Rogers. In my view, the chapter fails to fully press the implications of post-structural critiques for the practice of psychology. Foucauldian critique surfaces the problematic self-centred assumptions of Rogerian views but can be equally applied to the tenets of "narrative therapy" as articulated by Besley. In other words, two main parts of the chapter, an exegesis of Foucault and a presentation of narrative therapy, stand separately from each other, lacking critical interaction. (c) Drummond's critical exposition of the knowledge economy is followed by an insightful, if somewhat romantic, vision of a way to escape its discontents through *care of the self* theorized by Foucault in his late works.

2009
A bilingual, open-access online journal *Aporia – The nursing journal* launched in the University of Ottawa, Canada, under the editorship of Dave Holmes.

Date from the earliest	Author, title, summary
24.2010	Trudy Rudge & Dave Holmes (Eds.) *Abjectly boundless: Boundaries, bodies and health work.*
	A collection of 16 chapters, 2 of which previously appeared as journal articles. The contributors mostly draw on J. Kristeva's notion of the abject. In addition, Foucault's work features prominently in the chapters by a Canadian nurse Holmes and an Australian A. Street (e.g. the notion of discourse).
25.2012	Christine Ceci, Kristín Björnsdóttir & Mary Ellen Purkis (Eds.) *Perspectives on care at home for older people.*
	This interdisciplinary, international (e.g. North America and Nordic countries) collection brings together scholars from nursing and the social sciences researching and theorizing in the field of critical ageing studies. The central problematic of the book, articulated in the context of ethnographic studies sensitive to the material and discursive practices of formal home care provision for the older people, is "the conditions of possibility for good care" (p. ix). Although the authors draw on various theoretical concepts such as Agamben's *"whatever singularities"* (Purkis, 2012, p. 26) and Mol's *logic of care* (Ceci, 2012, p. 92), Foucault's understanding of power, governmentality, the medical gaze, and the conditions of possibility underlie several arguments made by the nurse contributors (i.e., the three editors and Latimer) and others.
26.2012	Dave Holmes, Trudy Rudge & Amélie Perron (Eds.) *(Re)thinking violence in health care settings: A critical approach.*
	A collection of 18 chapters (some are previously published papers and conference presentations) by authors from nursing, communication studies, justice studies, and rhetoric, from the United Kingdom, Australia, the United States, and Canada. To analyse violence, contributors variously draw on the work of P. Bourdieu, J. Butler, M. Foucault, B. Latour, and S. Žižek among other theorists.
	Penny Powers, who studied with David Allen at the University of Washington (refer to Table A2) reports on a Foucault-informed discourse-analytic study.
	Foucault is also cited by Canadians Holmes and his former students at the University of Ottawa: St-Pierre, Jacob, and O'Byrne. These scholars deploy the notion of power, both biopolitical power (as in Holmes and Murray's [2011] critique of the behaviour modification programs in forensic psychiatry) and disciplinary power with its components of hierarchical observation, examination, and normalizing judgements, for example, at play in the instances of intra/inter-professional aggression (St-Pierre & Holmes, 2010) or the public health practices in the domain of sexual health nursing assessment (Holmes & O'Byrne, 2006).
27.2013	Anette Forss, Christine Ceci & John Drummond (Eds.) *Philosophy of nursing: 5 questions.*
	From the 24 contributors, 6 – David Allen (United States), Drummond (Scotland), Holmes (Canada), Purkis (Canada), Rolfe (United Kingdom), and Rudge (Australia) – explain why they find post-structural theory and/or Foucault useful.
	Also included in this volume is Patricia Benner who cites Foucault's *The Birth of the Clinic* (refer to Table A2).

(Continued)

Date from the earliest	Author, title, summary
28.2013	Gary Rolfe *The university in dissent: Scholarship in the corporate university.* The first part of the book is an exegesis of Bill Reading's *The University in Ruins* (1996), an analysis of the demise of "the university of culture" and the rise of "the university of excellence," where *excellence* is an empty signifier easily accommodated to the market imperatives. Rolfe's 120-page book is saturated with references to Adorno, Badiou, Barthes, Deleuze and Guattari, Derrida, Foucault, Habermas, Heidegger, Lyotard, Wittgenstein, Žižek, and other philosophers. Parts of this book have earlier appeared in print as journal papers.
29.2013	Michael Traynor *Nursing in context: Policy, politics, profession.* Although possibly designed as an introductory text for nursing students in the United Kingdom, this little book is useful for a much wider audience of nurse readers. A unique feature of this book is its non-romantic representation of nursing practice embedded in the context of policy and inter-professional organizational workings. Foucault's notion of governmentality informs selected parts in the text.
30.2014	Dave Holmes, Jacob Jean-Daniel & Amélie Perron (Eds.) *Power and the psychiatric apparatus: Repression, transformation and assistance.* Foucault, Deleuze and Guattari, Goffman, and Szasz are central theoretical influences in this edited collection. Includes chapters by the editors themselves as well as by Paula J. Kagan (United States), Jem Masters, Rudge, and Sandra West (Australia), and Thomas Foth (Holmes's colleague and a former student).
31.2015	Amélie Perron & Trudy Rudge *On the politics of ignorance in nursing and healthcare: Knowing ignorance.* The authors start with an overview of a relatively new field of ignorance studies spanning sociology, epistemology, and education. Throughout the text, the authors cite nursing feminist, postcolonial, and post-structural scholars as well as contemporary sociologists (Giddens, Bauman, Beck, Latour) and French theorists (Foucault, Kristeva). The authors discuss what they call "nonknowledges" in nursing and health work including uncertainty, abjection, denial, deceit, and taboo. They explore how managerial practices perpetuate ignorance in health care organizations.
32.2015	Davina Allen *The invisible work of nurses: Hospitals, organizations and healthcare.* This manuscript is based on the ethnography of contemporary nursing practice in the United Kingdom. The author articulates translational mobilization theory to describe nurses' organizing work. Allen is not a "Foucauldian" scholar, but we find an occasional reference to Foucault's *The Birth of the Clinic.*

Index

Note 1: Page numbers followed by "n" indicate a note on the corresponding page.
Note 2: Appendix material is not included in the Index.

Abbott, A. 40 *see also* professionalization; sociology
actor network theory 132; *see also* Latour, B.
adaptation model (Roy) *see* Roy's adaptation model *Advanced Qualitative Research for Nursing* 133n2; *see also* Latimer, J.; qualitative research
Advances in Nursing Science (ANS) 7, 25, 31, 32–33n1, 53n11, 60, 61, 76n1, 103, 120, 133n1; frameworks and models 84–85; French theory in 93–94; "Fundamental Patterns of Knowing in Nursing" 84; notions of the person, empowerment, and experience 91–94; postmodern and post-structural work survey 87–94; practice-oriented models 86; *see also* Chinn, P.L.
Allen, D. 3, 52n5, 53n8, 69, 130, 131
Allen, D. G. 22, 27, 94, 95, 134n4; *see also* enclave groupAlthusser 26
American exceptionalism, critique of 125–126
American nursing science 2, 8, 38, 52n2, 60, 83, 84, 95; and disciplinary nursing knowledge 5–7, 12, 39, 42, 48–49, 60, 122, 128; formation of 40–42; logical positivism/positivism 39; logical positivist beliefs 46–50; logical positivist conception of theory 42–46; use of the term philosophy in 28–30; significance of Risjord's criticism of 38–39; *see also* American nursing theory; matrix; unique nursing knowledge/science/theory
American nursing theory 1–2, 5–7, 8–12, 60, 62, 95, 121–122; ANS 82–94;

capitalist ethos of 126–127; criticisms of 38–53, 102–116; disciplinary theory-building 3; emergence of 123–125; immunity to continental philosophy criticism 123–127; double-helix structure 122; NSQ 73–75; postmodern and post-structural ideas in 58–76; practice theory in 53n8; theorizing 13n1, 127–128; theory development 13n1; *see also* logical positivist conception of science/theory; matrix
analytic philosophy 14n8, 21
anti-humanism 9, 20, 23, 24, 29, 131; *see also* Foucault, M.; post-structuralism
Aporia 32n1, 105; *see also* Holmes, D.
Arendt, H. 25
Ashley, J. A. 85; *see also* Advances in Nursing Science (ANS)
Australia: nurses 124; nursing education 124; nursing models and theory in 124–125; scholars from 4
Avant, K. C. 96

Barrett, E. 74
Barthes 26
Benner, P. 106
biomedicine 22, 89, 108
Bjornsdottir, K. 6, 7
Bluhm, R. L. 14n7
borrowed theory/interdisciplinarity, caution toward 3–4, 25, 48, 49–51, 53n9, 73, 75, 122; acceptance/reformulation of 29, 50, 73; ANS welcoming of 85–86; *see also* logical positivism/logical empiricism
Bournes, D. 66
Brown, C. 33n6, 133n1

Butler, J. 12, 29, 93; matrix of intelligibility 15n11
Buus, N. 103

Canadian Association for the History of Nursing conference 30
Canadian nursing: nursing education 124; theory in nursing education 1–7
capitalism 33n6
capitalist ethos 124, 126–127
care of the self 93, 120; see also Foucault, M.; Nelson, S.
caring science/theory 4–5, 71, 76, 126; see also Watson, J. Carper, B. 47, 84, 122; see also Advances in Nursing Science (ANS)
Cassandra 85; see also Chinn, P. L.
Chapman, G. 24, 32n1
Cheek, J. 133n1, 133n2; see also qualitative research
Chinn, P. L. 5, 74, 83, 85, 90, 96, 97n2, 97n6, 122; see also Advances in Nursing Science (ANS)
Cixous, H. 23
Clarke, L. 26, 51n1, n2
classification/categories, limitations of 20, 132–133
Cloyes, K. G. 87, 93, 95; see also enclave group
Cody, W. K. 73, 75, 128
concept 2, 46–47, 50, 86–87
Contemporary Nursing Knowledge: Analysis and Evaluation of Nursing Models and Theories 48; see also Fawcett, J.
continental philosophy 21–25, 29; American nursing theory's immunity to criticisms of 123–127; classification of 25–27; as scientific method substitute, Gortner's critique of 63–64, 75; see also borrowed theory; Frankfurt school of critical theory; hermeneutics; phenomenology; post-structuralism; postmodernism
critical theory see Frankfurt school of critical theory; Freire, P.; Habermas, J.
Crowley, D. 47

Deleuze, G. 23
Derrida, J. 23, 25, 26
Dickoff, J. 49, 53n8
Dilthey, W. 43
discourse 10, 11, 23, 24, 30, 93, 109; see also Foucault, M.
Doering, L. 87

Donaldson, S. K. 44, 47
Drevdahl, D. 87, 92, 95; see also enclave group
Drummond, J. S. 120
Dzurec, L. 25, 64, 86, 87, 121

Edwards, S. D. 33n7
Ellis, R. 49, 53n8
emancipatory nursing practice 97n6, 134n4; see also Advances in Nursing Science (ANS); Chinn, P.L.
empiricism see logical positivism/logical empiricism
empowerment, patient 92–93; see also Powers, P.
enclave group 4, 94–96, 120, 123, 126; see also Allen, D. G.; Cloyes, K. G.; Drevdahl, D.; Hardin, P. K.; Phillips, D.; Powers, P.; Thompson, J.
episteme 2, 11–12; discursive and non-discursive element 11; epistemological unconscious 15n11; see also Foucault, M.
ethnomethodology 52n5, 53n8; see also sociology

Fawcett, J. 2, 5, 12, 25, 46–49, 53n11, 71, 83, 84, 122
Feigl, H. 45
feminism/feminists 63, 85; American nursing feminist discourse 90; critical social feminism 90; cultural 90; emancipation of women 88–89; feminist discourse 86, 88, 90; feminist writers 63; French feminist post-structuralists 23; liberal 90; postmodern perspective 87, 89; theorists 89; theorizing 85; see also Advances in Nursing Science (ANS); Butler, J.; Cassandra
Forss, A. 130
"Foucault and Nursing: A History of the Present" 105; see also Gastaldo, D.; Holmes, D.
Foucault, M. 2, 4, 6, 9, 10, 14n10, 20, 23–25, 29, 67, 73, 75, 86, 93, 123; episteme and the conditions of possibility 11–12; see also anti-humanism; post-structuralism
Francis, B. 33n6
Frankfurt school of critical theory 20, 22, 23, 29, 31, 33n2; see also Habermas, J.
Freire, P. 86, 88
French theory 7, 9, 13, 26, 30, 73, 82, 96, 114–115, 129; in American nursing 96; in ANS 93–94; nursing and

27–30; *see also* continental philosophy; postmodernism; post-structuralism

Freshwater, D. 131

Freud 26, 125

"Fundamental Patterns of Knowing in Nursing" 47, 84; *see also* Carper, B.

Gadamer, H-G. 21, 95

Gadow, S. 106, 116n5

Garrett, B. 26, 123

Gastaldo, D. 103, 124

gaze: clinical 88, 106, 109, 110, 120; medical 24, 106, 112; nursing 24; *see also* Foucault, M.

Genealogy of Care of the Sick: Nursing, Holism, and Pious Practice, A 111; *see also* Nelson, S.

German critical theory *see* Frankfurt school of critical theory

Gibbs, J. P. 45; *see also* sociology

Giddens, A. 127; *see also* sociology

Glazer, S. 26, 73, 77n10, 123

Goffman 26; *see also* sociology

Gortner, S. R. 59–64, 75, 76n3

Gunter, L. M. 53n8

Habermas, J. 20, 22, 27, 86, 88, 94, 95

Hage, J. 45; *see also* sociology

Haraway, D. 132

Harding, S. 76n3, 90, 97n4, 125

Hardin, P. K. 95; *see also* enclave group

Heidegger, M. 21

Hempel, C. 45, 95

Henderson, V. 41

hermeneutics 7, 22, 62–64, 94, 95, 106

Hiraki, A. 22

holism *see* holistic nurse

holistic nurse 108–109; American theoretical nursing 113; Christian ethos 111–112; described 111; ethos of agape 112; humanist philosophy 112; model of nursing care 109; nursing theory 108, 113–114; transcendent caring moments 113; valorization 112–113; *see also* Nelson, S.

Holmes, D. 103, 105, 124

Hospitals, Paternalism, and the Role of the Nurse 85; *see also* Ashley, J. A.

humanbecoming theory 3, 76n4, 77n6, 97n2; *see also* Parse, R.R.

humanism 4, 12, 20, 24, 29, 62, 69, 106, 110, 111, 112–113, 131

humanistic ideals of American nursing theory 29, 106, 111–114

humanistic values 70–71; of caring 62; in nursing theory 20–21, 62; *see also* American nursing theory; holistic nurse; nurse-patient relationships

Husserl, E. 21, 43

ideal vision of nursing 128

Image 95

In Search of Nursing Science 64

In Sickness and In Health (ISIH) group 27, 105, 121

"Intelligent Nursing: Accounting for Knowledge as Action in Practice" 6; *see also* Bjornsdottir, K.; Purkis, M. E.

International Critical and Feminist Perspectives in Nursing conferences 4

International Journal of Nursing Studies (IJNS) 116n6, 133n1

International Philosophy of Nursing Society (IPONS) 3, 27, 120–121

Irigaray, L. 23

Jameson, F. 33n6

Johnson, B. M. 96

Johnson, D. E. 48

Jonas-Simpson, C. 97n2

Journal of Advanced Nursing (JAN) 7, 24, 30, 31, 32–33n1, 33n5, 95, 103, 105, 116n6, 120, 124, 133n1

Journal of Clinical Nursing (JCN) 32–33n1

Journal of Psychiatric and Mental Health Nursing (JPMHN) 32n1

Kagan, P. N. 97n6, 134n4

Kermode, S. 33n6, 133n1

Kikuchi, J. F. 51n1

Kim, H. S. 47, 130

knowing the patient, critical analysis 109–110, 115; *see also* May, C. R.

Kollak, I. 130

Kramer, M. K. 96, 97n2, 97n6

Kristeva, J. 23, 26

Kuhn, T. 15n11, 68, 95, 124

Lacan, J. 29, 71, 90

Latimer, J. 27, 130, 133n2, 134n2

Latour, B. 26; *see also* actor network theory

Laudan, L. 95

Lawler, J. 124

Lees, G. 24, 32n1

Lenz, E. R. 53n10

Leonard, R. C. 42, 49, 53n8

Levinas, E. 20, 27

Lévi-Strauss, C. 23, 26

Liaschenko 39, 69, 110, 115n1, 116n4, 133n1
lived experience *see* phenomenology
logical positivism/logical empiricism 14n7, 39–41, 43, 52n3; described 43; received view of theory 40–41; *see also* logical positivist conception of science/theory
logical positivist conception of science/ theory 8, 14n7; borrowed theory 49–50; concept 2, 46–47, 50, 86–87; definitions of 45–47; empiricism 43; metaparadigm 6, 14n7, 38, 41, 48, 51, 65, 66, 87, 92, 114, 121, 128; paradigm 3, 6, 7, 14n7, 22, 25, 38, 51, 60, 62, 63, 64, 66, 68–69, 70, 71, 72, 75, 76, 76n2, 77n6, 85, 86, 87, 121, 122; philosophers of science and nurses 44–45; pyramid image of 14, 38, 39, 46, 51, 65, 66; structure of nursing knowledge 11, 14n5, 25, 48–49, 51, 97n1, 130; terminology 42–43; value-free or value-laden 46–48; verification principle 43–44; Vienna Circle 43–44; criticisms of *see* Paley; Risjord; Thompson
Lyotard, J-F. 23, 26, 67, 127

Marx 26, 125
matrix: disciplinary 15n11; heterosexual 12; intellectual 7, 8; of intelligibility 8, 12, 38, 130; *see also* Butler, J; American nursing science; American nursing theory; unique nursing knowledge/ science/theory
May, C. R. 27, 102, 107–109, 115, 116n6, 116n7
medical model 59, 87, 91, 130
Meleis, A. I. 30, 39, 96, 110
Merleau-Ponty, M. 21
metanarratives: Reed, P. and 67–70, 76n5; postmodernism's suspicion toward 24, 67; Watson, J. 73–74
metaparadigm 6, 14n7, 38, 41, 48, 51, 65, 66, 87, 92, 114, 121, 128
methodological considerations 8–11, 31n1, 97n5, 115n3, 133n1, 133n2
Mitchell, G. J. 66, 75, 128
models in nursing 12, 44, 53n11, 69, 84–85
modernism 24, 67; *see also* neomodernism
morality 20, 29–30, 72; teaching moral values in nursing 113
moral realism 33n7

Nagel, E. 45
"Necessity for and Evolution of Multiple Paradigms for Nursing Research:

A Poststructuralist Perspective"64–65; *see also* Dzurec, L.
Nelson, S. 23, 27, 30, 102, 111–115, 116n5, 120, 122, 124, 129, 130
neomodernism 67, 69, 70, 76; *see also* Reed, P. G.
Newman, M. A. 46, 67, 72
New Zealand 4, 124
Nietzsche, F. 23, 29, 90
Nortvedt, P. 33n7
nurse-patient relationships 105–106, 116n7; American nursing theories 110–111; authentic relationships 109; condition of possibility 110; contextual attitude 107–108; dyadic interaction 107–108; holism 108; holistic practice 108–109; human life in postmodern times 106; knowing the patient 109–110, 115; notion of power/knowledge 108; relational 106; social theory 110; talk context in 109; technocratic attitude 107, 108
Nurse Researcher (NR) 32n1
"Nursing as Means of Governmentality" 105; *see also* Gastaldo, D.; Holmes, D.
nursing education 124–125; critical theoretical nursing discourse 130–132; curricular categories, limitations of 132–133; nursing practice in theoretical accounts 127–130
Nursing Ethics (NE) 27, 32n1
Nursing Inquiry (NI) 7, 30, 31, 32–33n1, 95, 103, 105, 120, 124, 133n1
Nursing Knowledge: Science, Practice, and Philosophy 9; *see also* Risjord, M.
Nursing Philosophy (NP) 7, 27, 30, 31, 32–33n1, 95, 103, 105, 120
Nursing Research 40, 41
nursing science *see* American nursing science; *also see* American nursing theory; Gortner, S.
Nursing Science Quarterly (NSQ) 7, 60, 66, 73–75, 97n2, 122
"Nursing's Syntax Revisited: A Critique of Philosophies Said to Influence Nursing Theories" 59–64; *see also* Gortner, S.
Nursing Theorists and Their Work 130

Obama, B. 125
Order of Things, The 11; *see also* Foucault, M.
Orem, D. 67, 95
Orlando, I. J. 71

Paley, J. 29, 72, 77n9
paradigm: in American nursing theory 3,
   6, 7, 14n7, 22, 25, 38, 51, 60, 62, 63,
   64, 66, 68–69, 70, 71, 72, 75, 76, 76n2,
   77n6, 85, 86, 87, 121, 122; Kuhnian
   15n11, 68, 76n2; criticisms of 59, 68,
   76n2, 93–110, 128, 133n1, 134n4
Parker, J. M. 6, 27, 120, 124
Parse, R. R. 3, 72, 73, 76n4, 77n6, 95;
   see also humanbecoming theory; *Nursing
   Science Quarterly (NSQ)*
patients: empowerment 92–93; nurse-
   patient relationship 105–111
patterns of knowing in nursing 3, 58, 84,
   97n1, 128, 130; *see also* Carper, B.; ways
   of knowing in nursing
Peplau, H. 71
Perron, A. 125, 134n4
person, notions of 91–92, 128; *see also*
   subject/subjectivity
Perspectives on Nursing Theory 14n5, 65;
   see also Reed. P. G.; Shearer, N. B. C.
*Perspectives on Philosophy of Science in
   Nursing* 64; *see also* Polifroni E. C.;
   Welch, M.
phenomenology 22; as lived experience
   22, 29; as research methodology 21–23,
   64
Phillips, D. 87, 93, 95; *see also* enclave
   group
philosophy of science 3, 9, 40–51, 84, 95,
   113; academic discipline of nursing in
   United States 124–125; anthology of
   121; metaphysical turn 62; paradigm 68,
   76n2; postmodern 64, 67; postpositivist
   53n10, 60
Polifroni, E. C. 64, 70, 74, 88
Porter, S. 22, 27, 104, 123
positivism *see* logical positivism/logical
   empiricism
*Postmodern and Poststructural Approaches to
   Nursing Research* 133n2; *see also* Cheek J.
postmodernism 6, 24, 123; classification
   troubles 25–27; continental philosophy
   24; criticisms of in nursing 26, 28,
   29–30, 33n6, 73, 77n10, 104, 123; in
   American nursing literature 58–59, 63,
   64–70, 71–74, 86–91, 92–94; and post-
   structuralism in non-American nursing
   literature 6–7, 14n5, 23, 103–116,
   120–122; *see also* post-structuralism;
   Sokal affair
"Postmodernism and Knowledge
   Development in Nursing" 70–75;
   see also Watson J.

Postmodern Nursing and Beyond 71, 72;
   see also Watson, J.
postpositivist philosophy of science 45, 49,
   53n10, 60, 62
post-structuralism 6, 23–24, 121;
   classification troubles 25–27;
   continental philosophy 23–24;
   discourses, primacy of language in
   23–24; *see also* anti-humanism;
   Foucault, M.; postmodernism
power 10, 11, 24, 74, 92, 106, 108–109;
   power/knowledge24, 25, 64, 67, 90, 93,
   103; *see also* Foucault, M.
"Power, Right, and Truth: Foucault's
   Triangle as a Model for Clinical Power"
   74; *see also* Polifroni E. C.
Powers, P. 87, 92, 93, 95; *see also* enclave
   group
practice: practice-based theory 49, 65–
   67, 69, 76n5; practice-guiding grand
   theory 66; practice-oriented models
   86; practice theory 42, 49, 53n8;
   nursing practice in American nursing
   theory 22, 28, 41, 46, 127–129;
   see also holistic nurse; nurse-patient
   relationships
professionalization 3, 108, 124; *see also*
   Abbott, A.
Purkis, M. E. 6, 7, 23, 106, 133n1
Putnam, H. 49
pyramid structure of American nursing
   theory/deductive-nomological 39, 46,
   53n7, 65, 66, 70, 86; *see also* logical
   positivism/logical empiricism; American
   nursing science; American nursing theory

qualitative research 20–22, 27, 104,
   132–133

Reed, P. G. 14n5, 59, 65–72, 74, 76n5,
   77n7, 88, 121, 122
"Relationship between Theory and
   Research, The: A Double Helix" 83;
   see also Fawcett, J.
religious nursing 111; *see also* holistic
   nurse; Nelson, S.
Research and Theory for Nursing Practice
   133n1
Research in Nursing and Health 61, 83
*Research, Truth, and Authority: Postmodern
   Perspectives on Nursing* 133n2; *see also*
   Rolfe, G.
Risjord, M. 8, 9, 12, 14n6, 14n7, 14n8,
   28, 38–40, 42–53, 58, 60, 65, 95, 113,
   114, 121, 122, 128, 130; *see also* logical

positivist beliefs in nursing science (Risjord)
Rogers, M. 66, 72, 95
Rolfe, G. 133n2
Rorty, R. 26, 67
Roy, C. 2, 47, 95, 97n6
Roy's adaptation model 2, 4; *see also* Roy, C.
Rudge, T. 27, 125, 133n1, 134n4

Sandelowski, M. 14n6, 116n9, 130
Saussure, F. 23, 26, 71
Schlotfeldt, R. M. 48
Scholarly Inquiry for Nursing Practice (SINP) 133n1
scientific theory *see* American nursing science; American nursing theory; logical positivism/logical empiricism; Risjord, M.
"Self," the 104; *see also* Foucault, M.; subject/subjectivity
self-reflective narratives/journaling 3, 29, 112; criticism of 23; reflexivity 131
Shearer, N. B. C. 14n5
Smith, D. 27, 76n3; *see also* sociology
Social Text see Sokal affair
sociology 1, 4, 26, 27, 30, 42, 45, 73, 107, 110; theory/theories 4, 110–111; *see also* Abbott, A.; ethnomethodology; Goffman; Gibbs, J. P.; Giddens, A.; Hage, J.; Smith, D.; Turner, J.
Sokal affair 123, 134n3; *see also* postmodernism, criticisms of in nursing
Street, A. F. 134n4
structure of nursing knowledge 5, 25, 48–49; *see also* Fawcett, J.
subject/subjectivity 4, 29, 92, 129; criticisms of 95–96; essential subject 104; Foucault's ideas on power and 104, 106; humanistic subject 106; the "Self" 104; *see also* anti-humanism

Theodoridis, K. 51n1
theoretical anti-humanism *see* anti-humanism

Theoretical Nursing: Development and Progress 110; *see also* Meleis A. I.
Thompson, J. L. 22, 77n10, 94, 95, 130; *also see* enclave group
Topaz, M. 74
Traynor, M. 27, 131
"Treatise on Nursing Knowledge Development for the 21st Century: Beyond Postmodernism" 65–70; *see also* Reed, P. G.
Turner, J. 45; *see also* sociology

unintelligible 6–7, 12, 38, 59, 102, 122–123, 128, 132; *see also* matrix
unique nursing knowledge/science/theory 3, 5, 7, 8, 25, 48, 59, 70, 72, 75, 76, 83, 115, 122, 123, 128–129; *see also* American nursing science; American nursing theory; matrix; Risjord, M.
United Kingdom (UK) 4, 5, 13; nursing education 124; scholars from 4

value-free/value laden, theory as 47–48
Van Orman Quine, V. 49
verification principle 43–44
Vienna Circle 43–44

Wald, F. S. 42, 49, 53n8
Walker, L. O. 46, 96
Watson Caring Science Institute website 126; *see also* Watson, J.
Watson, J. 4, 59, 64, 70–75, 77n8, 88, 121, 126, 127; *see also* caring science/theory
ways of knowing in nursing 84, 87–89, 97n2, 122; emancipatory 123; multiple 87
Webber, P. B. 96
Webster, G. 39
Welch, M. 64, 70
Western Journal of Nursing Research, The 61, 83
Wied, S. 110

Printed in the United States
by Baker & Taylor Publisher Services